MW01290211

PARENTS WHO KILLED

THEIR CHILDREN

ISBN-13 978-1494787066
ISBN-10 1494787067

Written by

RJ Parker

RJ PARKER PUBLISHING, INC.
Published in the United States of America

Edited by Deb Hartwell
(Hartwell Editing)
Cover design by Jacqueline Cross

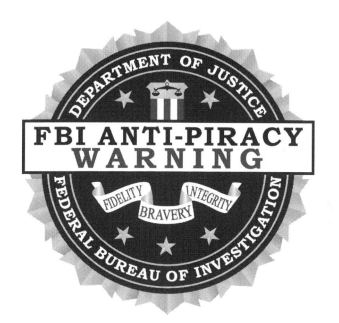

Table of Contents

8

Prologue

We consider mothers to hold the highest status in our lives. For a son, there is no greater being on this planet than his mother. She gives birth to the child, cares for him when he is in his most vulnerable state, unable to eat or drink, and she feeds him her own milk. Suffice it to say, the role of a mother is one that cannot be explained properly in words. What she does for her child is the real example of true love; she does everything for him without ever wanting anything back.

However, throughout the history of time, we have learned that there is no end to the cruelty of mankind. We commit the most heinous crimes, sometimes the most unthinkable acts and yet, we never seem to learn. The bond between a mother and her child is a sacred one. The powers of love, care, and trust that bind this bond are so strong that it is a virtually unbreakable bond. A mother cannot lose her child, and if she does, she is heartbroken. Similarly, a child cannot lose his mother. If he does, through any incident, he will forever miss her. Children look up to their mothers, considering them to be a shelter for them. The minute she gives birth, the status of an ordinary woman is elevated to a sacred one: that of a mother. Certain expectations are attached to her role; her responsibilities increase and in virtually every religion, the position of a mother is an exalted one. Throughout our lives, we have read stories of the bravery of mothers to support and help their children. We have read of single mothers who bore all of the hardships of life just so that they could provide for their children. You might have heard of numerous women out there who have even sold their bodies just so that they could earn enough to support their young ones. However, the stories you are about to read are true, albeit very different than what we have grown up believing about our mothers. It is a sad instance of how deep one can fall as a victim to drugs, addictions, and insanity.

The term *filicide* is a funny one. Sometimes, I doubt whether this word should even exist in the dictionary or not. Filicide is the killing of a child by his or her own parent. Can man be capable of doing such a thing? We grow up being loved and adored by our parents. Sure, not everybody has the perfect life. Some children are born and raised in broken families, having to move from one place to another, switching houses between father and mother. Sometimes, things are worse: the parents may be drunk and abusive and may use violence as a means of venting out their frustrations, beating the children and abusing their rights as parents.

Even though bad parenting is a pretty big issue, most parents still show undying love for their children. And that is how it should be, of course. We have all received the occasional spanking from our parents, yet biologically, the mind of a child is engineered in such a way that he only finds relief, security, and safety when he is in the arms of his mother. This is how it's supposed to be; it feels natural and automated. Even if you take a cursory look at the news, you will find that the number of stories regarding struggling single mothers who are willing to go to any extent to support their children and help them in any way possible are much higher. Stories regarding the abuse of children by their own mothers are obviously fewer in comparison, and that is what our society is like; it's how our minds are engineered to be.

Whenever we hear about instances of cruelty from parents on their children, we are often confused. Why would a parent hit his or her own offspring? Or abuse them? More often than not, the blame goes to their mental conditions. Most parents often become mentally unstable whenever things tend to get out of hand. Imagine a single mother, tired of fighting with society for herself and her child, jobless, trying to support two people. How long would you expect her to keep it together? Often times, the parents release their frustration on the child, and as a child grows, she eventually realizes that. Yet, it is a heartless, shameful act to subject one's own child to cruelty. The stories that follow go against everything we have been taught and have learned. We perceive mothers to be the epitome of care and support, yet mankind teaches us cruel lessons.

Filicide

Filicide is the intended act of a parent killing his or her own child. The act is also regarded as an offence since it amounts to murder. To most of society, filicide appears very unnatural and inhumane, yet a small percentage of parents exist who do kill their offspring. Many researchers and scholars have associated these tragedies as being caused by domestic violence. According to Jill Proudfoot of the Auckland Safer Homes, threats of violence are a common occurrence in relationships and it is the use of such threats that keeps a woman in a given relationship. However, this does not mean that all parents who commit filicide have mental problems.

The Causes of Filicide

Researchers point to numerous possible reasons behind incidents of filicide. Some of them are as follows:

Altruism

In this instance, a parent murders his or her child in order to end some form of suffering that the child may be experiencing. The suffering of the child may be in form of incapacity both of the mind or body. A parent may thus become so depressed by the condition of the child and cannot stand the idea of leaving the child to suffer, hence reasoning that ending the child's life is the only way of helping. Other times the child may not be really suffering but exhibits the signs of suffering or incapacitation.

Acute Psychosis

In some instances, a parent commits

filicide because of a defect of reasoning or because the parent is mentally ill. This mainly happens when there is no reasonable explanation to account for the murder of the child. In the 2001 case of Andrea Yates, who was accused of drowning her children in a bathtub, she was found to be laboring from insanity and found not guilty for killing her five children. She psychically believed that upon maturity, her babies will come to harm and that she was helping by saving them from that harm.

An Unwanted Child

This is quite self-explanatory. If a parent does not like or love his or her child and feels that the child is a big drawback to the goals of his or her life, this may push the parent to get rid of the child so as to be set free.

Child Maltreatment

Many reported filicides are caused as a result of child maltreatment. This essentially involves a tragic accident that occurs during child abuse. The parent may think that he is punishing the child and in the process goes too far such that grievous harm is caused or at times instant deaths.

Filicide caused as a result of spousal revenge is rare, as not many reasonable parents would willingly harm their children to get back at their spouse. However, there are some instances when parents kill their children for revenge. Sometimes it is referred to as **Medea Syndrome**, which is translated from Greek mythology. In the myth, Medea murders her child so as to inflict suffering to her husband, Jason, who was alleged to be having an affair. There are other causes that are independent of the above; a good example is probably the famous case of Susan Smith who was accused in 1994 of drowning her two children in a lake. In her hearing, she pleaded insanity but was sentenced to life imprisonment when the court found out that she had murdered her children because the man she wanted to be with did not want children.

According to experts, these parents usually don't understand the consequences of what they are doing during the act. It is also clear that in order to evade such tragedies in the future, we should focus on the prevention. This can be done through family and friends being there for troubled parents, enabling them to deal maturely with the stress by getting help.

Chapter 1: Andrea Yates

Background

The youngest of five children, Andrea Yates was born Andrea Pia Kennedy on July 2, 1964, in Hallsville, Texas. Her mother, Jutta Karin Koehler, was a German immigrant and her father, Andrew Emmett Kennedy, was the son of Irish parents.

As a teen, Andrea suffered from several bouts of depression and was bulimic. At the age of 17, she had spoken to a friend about suicide. Yet, in 1982 she graduated from Milby High School in Houston, Texas with honors as class valedictorian, captain of the swim team, and an officer in the National Honor Society.

Andrea went on to complete her

nursing degree from the University of Texas School of Nursing at the University of Houston Campus in 1986. She then became a Registered Nurse at the highly regarded University of Texas M.D. Anderson Cancer Center in Houston, Texas.

After graduation, Andrea made her home at the Sunscape Apartments in Houston, Texas. There, in 1989, she met her future husband, Russell "Rusty" Yates. They soon moved in together, and on April 17, 1993, they married. Rusty was an acquaintance of Preacher Michael Peter Woroniecki, whom he met while attending Auburn University. Woroniecki's church condemned the couple for their Christian lifestyle and believed that their future children would be doomed to hell for their parents' sins. Woroniecki's church also believed in the "Quiverfull lifestyle," which means that married couples should have as many children as possible.

On February 26, 1994, Andrea gave birth to a son, Noah. Soon after, the Yates family decided to relocate to Florida where Rusty had accepted a job offer. The family settled into a small trailer home in Seminole, Florida. While there, Andrea gave birth to a second son, John, on December 15, 1995. The stay in Seminole, Florida was brief and the family relocated back to Houston shortly after John's birth. On September 13, 1997, Andrea gave birth to yet another son named Paul. Shortly after his birth, she became very depressed. On February 15, 1999, she gave birth to a fourth son, Luke. This marked the beginning of Andrea's psychosis.

On June 16, 1999, Andrea had her first mental breakdown. Rusty found his wife chewing on her fingers and shaking uncontrollably. She was then admitted to the hospital and placed on antidepressants. Shortly after her release, she held a knife to her own neck and pleaded with her husband to let her die. She was readmitted to the hospital and given a cocktail of different medications. One of these medications was Haldol, an antipsychotic drug. With this combination of drugs, Andrea's condition improved and she was released. She seemed to be stable, but in July of 1999, she suffered another nervous breakdown, followed by two suicide attempts. She went on to be hospitalized two more times that summer. During her treatment, she was diagnosed with postpartum psychosis.

Andrea's first psychiatrist advised her to not have any more children, as this would certainly lead to future psychotic episodes. Against the advice of her doctor, Andrea conceived her fifth child. She stopped taking the medication Haldol in March of 2000. On November 30, 2000, her fifth child, a daughter named Mary, was born.

"Woe to the bad mother. Children end up sinful if the mother doesn't take a switch to them." – Tract by Preacher Woroniecki

The morning of June 20, 2001 began as usual in the Yates' home. Andrea got out of bed at approximately 8:10 a.m., and all of the children were awake. They were sitting around the breakfast table eating their cereal as they did every morning. Rusty left for work at around 9:00 a.m.; nothing seemed out of the ordinary.

Shortly after her husband left the house, Andrea wandered into the bathroom where she filled the tub with water about three inches from the top rim. Mary, then six months old, sat on the bathroom floor.

Paul came into the bathroom and asked, "Mommy, are we gonna take a bath?" He asked the question a second time when his mother did not answer. Andrea then took three-year-old Paul and placed him face down into the water. There was only a brief struggle due to his young age. Once she knew he was no longer breathing, she took his lifeless body into the bedroom and laid it on the bed. The exact procedure was repeated with two-year-old Luke and then five-year-old John. Mary sat on the floor crying as her mother drowned her brothers. Andrea then picked Mary up and took her towards the water. She held her baby under the water face down until she was motionless and left her body floating in the tub.

Andrea then called for seven-year-old Noah to come to the bathroom. She knew he would put up the biggest struggle, as he was the oldest of the children. Noah walked in and saw Mary's body in the tub. He asked, "Mommy, what's wrong with Mary?" and then immediately tried to get away from his mother. He ran down the hall, but he was unable to escape. Andrea grabbed him and forced him into the water. Noah struggled all he could; he even came up for air a few times before he died. She left Noah's body in the water and removed Mary's. She walked to the master bedroom and placed her daughter's body on the bed along with the bodies of Paul, Luke, and John, all of which were covered with a sheet.

Shortly after drowning her five children, Andrea called 911 speaking in a calm and unemotional voice.

911 Dispatcher: What's your name?
Andrea Yates: Andrea Yates
911 Dispatcher: What's the problem?
Andrea Yates: Um, I just need him to come.
911 Dispatcher: Is your husband there?
Andrea Yates: No.
911 Dispatcher: Well, what's the problem?
Andrea Yates: I need him to come.
911 Dispatcher: I need to know why we're coming, ma'am. Is he there standing next to you?
Andrea Yates: No.
911 Dispatcher: She?
Andrea Yates: Pardon me?
911 Dispatcher: Are you having a disturbance? Are you ill or what?
Andrea Yates: Um, yes, I'm ill.
911 Dispatcher: Do you need an ambulance?
Andrea Yates: No, I need a police officer. Yeah, send an ambulance.
911 Dispatcher: What's the problem?
Andrea Yates: Um?
911 Dispatcher: Hello?
Andrea Yates: I just need a police officer.

She did not sound out of breath as she spoke, yet portions of the 911 recording indicated that heavy breathing could be heard. Shortly after, she called her husband at work and told him he needed to come home. He questioned her repeatedly, but all she told him was, "It is time."

There was a knock at the door. The police had arrived and Andrea simply stated, "I killed my kids." When the police asked her where the children were, she led them to the master bedroom. One of the officers noticed a small arm protruding from under the sheet. When he pulled it back, he observed the bodies of four small children. Another officer discovered Noah's body in the tub. They asked Andrea for consent to search the house and she agreed.

Andrea's clothing was wet and her hair was matted. Clothes were gathered from the bedroom for her to change into. There was no female officer with them, so they planned to take the dry clothing to the police station. They only spoke to her for a brief amount of time before the investigation ensued.

The officers then began taking photographs. Photos were taken in the hallway, where one of the officers had noticed small footprints upon arrival at the house. The carpet was soaked and 9 inches of water remained in the tub. An array of medications was found in the kitchen, including Effexor, Remeran, Wellbutrin, and Resperidol, which is classified as an antipsychotic medication. The cereal bowls on the table remained as the children had left them after eating breakfast that morning.

When later asked why she killed her children, Andrea answered, "It was not because of anything they had done or because I was mad at them. They just weren't developing correctly, and I am a bad mother." Her only question after giving her statement was, "When will my trial be?"

Yates' Trials

On September 22, 2001, a jury deliberated for more than eight hours to find that Andrea Yates was mentally competent to stand trial. Her religious beliefs about Satan and her profound history of mental illness would be challenged when her murder trial began on February 18, 2002.

Andrea pleaded not guilty by reason of insanity in the deaths of Noah and John and in a second charge for the death of Mary, but not for the deaths of Paul and Luke. In Texas, anyone convicted of multiple murders or the killing of an infant is eligible for the death penalty. According to Texas law, to successfully assert the insanity defense, attorneys must prove that at the time of the crime, "the actor, as a result of severe mental disease or defect, did not know that his conduct was wrong."

George Parnham, Andrea Yates' defense attorney, addressed the jury of eight women and four men. His question to them was, "How does a mother who has given birth, who has nurtured, who has protected, and who has loved the five children that she brought into this world, interrupt their lives?"

The defense team had several expert witnesses that addressed the mental illness known as postpartum psychosis. This is a condition when, if left untreated, the mother and child are at great risk of harm. The defense also addressed Andrea's suicide attempts, eating disorders, religious beliefs, and thoughts of the particular church led by Michael Woroniecki. The defense suggested that these types of beliefs and materials provided by the church were dangerous to someone like Andrea Yates.

Psychiatric observations conducted on Andrea showed that she was in a constant battle with Satan. She believed Satan was always nearby. While she did not believe she was possessed by Satan at the time of the murders, she admitted to feeling his presence. She claimed that once she was arrested, Satan was inside of her. Andrea also interpreted three scabs on her head as being the three 6s, or the marks of Satan. She had a habit of picking the scabs and pulling out the hair over the area, which inevitably exposed them. Andrea thought this was a sign for her to reveal the marks on her head and the manner in which Satan meant for her to interpret them.

Dr. Saeed, Andrea's prescribing physician, also testified. He described her as being, at times, unable to talk, unable to narrate, and unable to give proper answers. He also testified that on June 4, 2001, she had been taken off anti-psychotic medications. By June 7 or 8, all anti-psychotic medications were eliminated from her body and on June 20, the inevitable tragedy happened.

The prosecution's opening statements to the jury focused primarily on the day of the murders. They wanted to make sure the jury understood completely that Andrea Yates was sane when she drowned her five children. They claimed that on the day of the murders, Andrea may have been mentally ill, but she still knew right from wrong. In the state of Texas, this would not be considered legally insane.

Prosecuting attorneys presented a witness that testified about the autopsy results. He claimed that the children died slow deaths. In an autopsy photograph of John, he was shown still clutching a strand of his mother's long, dark hair. Noah's arms were shown raised above his head, his small fists in a permanent clenched position. His knees were bent, and he was stiff due to the extreme exertion on his body at the time of death. He had deep internal bruising, cuts, nail scratches, and round bruises on his joints, indicating the strong pressure from his mother's fingertips. These results showed that Noah fought the hardest to stay alive. Mary's autopsy revealed that she had much less bruising than her brothers. However, she had significant bruising on the back of her head from being forced under the water for several minutes.

The prosecution presented forensic psychiatrist Dr. Park Dietz as an expert witness. Dr. Dietz is nationally known for his authority on the Jeffrey Dahmer and Unabomber cases and was the only health expert to testify for the prosecution. Dr. Dietz was also a consultant for the TV show, *Law & Order*.

During his testimony, Dr. Dietz stated that shortly before the Yates' murders, an episode of *Law & Order* aired in which a woman who was suffering from postpartum depression drowned her children and was acquitted by reason of insanity. Other witnesses testified that Yates watched the television series regularly. This suggested to the jury that Yates had seen this particular episode and used it to plan and plot the murders of her five children.

There was just one problem with Dr. Dietz's recollection of this particular *Law & Order* episode: it never existed. Dr. Dietz soon realized that he had made a serious factual error. He decided that his recollection was incorrect. He had mistakenly meshed two episodes of *Law & Order* into one. One episode was based on the Susan Smith case. She was the mother who strapped her two children into car seats and drove the car into a lake. The other episode was based on Amy Grossberg and Melissa Drexler, two teen moms that were charged with discarding their newborn babies.

Dr. Dietz sent a letter to prosecutors explaining his mistake and offering to return to Houston to correct the error at his own expense. His letter, however, was never introduced as evidence.

After a Texas jury deliberated for three and a half hours in March of 2002, they found Andrea Yates guilty of capital murder. The jury showed her mercy and she was sentenced to life in prison without parole.

Andrea Yates' attorney filed an appeal on April 30, 2004, questioning the prosecution's testimony of Dr. Park Dietz. This would challenge the constitutionality of Texas's insanity law, which makes it nearly impossible for a defendant to hold a successful insanity defense. The Texas Court of Appeals reversed Andrea's convictions on January 6, 2005, due to the false testimony given by Dr. Dietz, and she was granted another trial.

On January 9, 2006, five years after she drowned her children, Andrea Yates again entered pleas of not guilty by reasons of insanity. The jury in her second trial was equally divided between six men and six women. The prosecution once again introduced Dr. Dietz's testimony, this time omitting any reference to a *Law & Order* episode. In his opinion, Andrea Yates knew the difference between right and wrong, and she had carried out well planned multiple murders. In this second trial, the same mental health records were introduced. Throughout the duration of the trial, expert witnesses would again chronicle her multiple stays in mental institutions, repeated suicide attempts, recurring hallucinations, and bouts with severe depression. The stresses of her marital life and times of living in the cramped quarters of a trailer with her husband and children were also addressed.

In a dramatic and unforeseen turnaround, Andrea Yates was found not guilty by reason of insanity on July 26, 2006. When her verdict was read, she lowered her head and quietly wept. Her family, as well as Rusty Yates, also cried. Andrea's defense attorney called the second verdict a "watershed event in the treatment of mental illness." Andrea's 2002 conviction triggered a debate over Texas's legal standard for mental illness, claiming the courts may not be treating postpartum depression seriously enough. This leaves the debate over whether or not, if it occurred again, a mother would receive sympathy for killing her children due to mental illness in the rigid and "tough on crime" state of Texas.

Conclusion

Andrea Yates was committed and placed in the maximum-security North Texas State Hospital in Vernon, Texas shortly after her 2006 verdict. In 2007, she was transferred to the Kerrville State Hospital in Kerrville, Texas. The hospital stands overlooking the Guadalupe River with no fences and no guards. However, patients are ordered to stay within the boundaries of the facility. Andrea was assigned one roommate, and she is allowed to participate in arts and crafts, gardening, and wood shop activities. She makes cards and aprons which she sells anonymously and donates the money to the Yates Children Memorial Fund. This organization, founded by Andrea's defense attorney George Parnham in 2002, was established to raise awareness about postpartum illness for the benefit of mother, child, and family.

In 2004, after an eleven-year marriage, Andrea's husband Rusty filed for divorce. He had been a major source of support for her, but the stress of her trials and the loss of his children had become too much for him. In the divorce agreement, Andrea was given $7000, her nursing chair that was used after giving birth, and the right to be buried in the family plot next to her five children. As of 2008, Rusty had remarried and has since welcomed a new baby into his life.

We can only speculate as to why the jury decided on such a different outcome in Andrea Yates' second trial. It is possible that the female jurors could relate to the challenges of being a caregiver, or the jury collectively may have focused more on Dr. Dietz's error in the *Law & Order* claim. The second jury took nearly four times longer to decide on a verdict than the original jury did in the first trial. They undoubtedly focused more on her severe psychosis and the evidence showing that she did not know her actions were "wrong" at the time of the murders. It is obvious to anyone reading through Andrea Yates' history of mental illness that she is a sad and very ill woman.

Some may believe that Andrea Yates "got away with murder." However, she will spend the rest of her life being treated and evaluated for signs of psychosis and most likely will be confined to a maximum-security mental facility. If her condition were to ever get better, or if she was released, she would most likely be an elderly woman by then.

One thing is for certain: Andrea Yates will forever live with the grim reality of not being able to watch her five children grow and enjoy the generations of grandchildren that would have followed.

Chapter 2: Darlie Routier

Background

Darlie Lynn Peck (Routier) was born in Altoona, PA on January 4, 1970. She was an attractive, hazel-eyed blonde that was doted on as a child. She was the first born of her father, Larry Peck, and mother, Darlie Peck. Her parents were divorced when she was very young. It was then that the domestic security she had known as a child was disrupted. One year later, her mother remarried after meeting a man named Dennis Stahl. As Darlie entered her teen years, the family relocated to Lubbock, Texas. This was a big change for her, but she and her two natural sisters, as well as her two stepsisters, got along well and managed to support each other during the transition. Eventually the Stahl's marriage dissolved, and her mother was again in search of a new husband.

Despite the changes that were occurring in her life, Darlie emerged from being a shy, young girl into a blossoming and sometimes "showy" teen, and boys were very attracted to the beautiful blonde. There was one boy in particular that was very interested in Darlie. His name was Darin Routier. As a teen he worked as a busboy at the local Western Sizzler restaurant along with Darlie's mother, "Mama Darlie." Her mother found him to be a very good-looking young man with high aspirations of his future. She insisted he would be a great catch for her oldest daughter. They were introduced and the two fell for each other immediately.

Darin and Darlie dated throughout high school. He was two years older than Darlie, and after graduation he decided to attend a technical college that required him to relocate from Lubbock to Dallas. Darlie, as well as mutual friends of the couple, decided to give Darin a going-away party. It was during the party that Darlie began showing signs of possessiveness and the more cunning nature that was lying underneath her innocent and sweet demeanor. She seemed angry that the attention was directed towards Darin and not her, and eventually decided to leave the party. Later that evening she returned to the party in a panic, falsely claiming someone had raped her. This gave Darlie the dose of attention that she had been craving.

In 1988, Darlie graduated from Monterey High School in Lubbock, Texas. It was then that she decided to join Darin in Dallas. He had been working as a technician for a computer chip company and eventually landed a job with the firm. The couple moved in together, saved their money, and married in August of 1988.

After an extravagant Jamaican honeymoon, the newlyweds decided to move into a new apartment near Darin's workplace. Within just a year, the couple had moved to a small house in Rowlett, Texas, where Darin started his own company called Testnec. His company tested computer circuit boards and he was able to operate out of the home.

On June 14, 1989, Darlie gave birth to the couple's first son. He was a healthy boy, and they named him Devon Rush. A few years later a second son, Damon Christian, arrived on February 19, 1991.

Darlie soon became a full time housewife and mother. With the success of Darin's company, they moved into the posh Dalrock Heights Addition of Rowlett, Texas. It was a quiet community and was known as a great place to raise a family. They lived in a large Georgian-style home, which included a sparkling Jaguar that graced the driveway. They also had purchased a twenty-seven-foot cabin cruiser that was kept in a marina on nearby Lake Ray Hubbard. Neighbors and friends of Darlie recalled her as being very flashy and sometimes gaudy. Her obsession with attention, money, and shopping began to detract her from her role as a mother. At times, neighbors complained that the children were unsupervised, and they believed Darlie seemed annoyed that she had to watch them.

On October 18, 1995, Darlie gave birth to yet another son named Drake. Soon after, she started showing signs of severe mood swings and rage. She was suffering from postpartum depression. Not helping matters, the couple's finances began to decline. Even though Testnec had successful profits, their income could not match the extravagant lifestyle they had grown to know. Ends suddenly could not be met.

Darlie soon fell into a deep depression. She eventually broke down to Darin and confessed to thoughts of suicide. Darin was able to console her, and things seemed to balance in their lives for a short time. However, one month later, life in this quiet and undisturbed neighborhood would take a very dark turn.

The Murders

In the early morning hours of June 6, 1996, Darlie Routier made a frantic call to the Rowlett Police Department 911 dispatch and said, "Somebody came in here...they broke in." The 911 operator responded with, "Ma'am?" assuming it was only a break in. Darlie followed with, "They just stabbed me and my children!"

During the 911 call, Darlie repeatedly mentioned her husband's name. His voice could be heard many times, but was mostly unintelligible. This would suggest that he was home at the time of the murders, sleeping upstairs along with their youngest son, Drake.

Darlie explained to the operator that she and her two boys, Devon and Damon, were sleeping downstairs. According to Darlie, she woke up to Damon saying, "Mommy, Mommy!" as he tugged on her nightshirt. It was then, she claimed, that she could see a man standing above her who proceeded to stab her, as well as her two young sons. She also explained how she fought until the man ran out into the garage and threw the knife down. During the 911 call, Darlie repeatedly said that they (her children) were "dying" or they were "dead." She told the operator that her husband had run down the stairs to help her, but he was apparently not aware of when the attack occurred. At one point during the call, Darlie became somewhat agitated about having to wait for the ambulance and said to the 911 operator, "I gotta just sit here forever...oh, my God."

There were many inconsistencies within the 911 call. Darlie repeatedly referred to the boys as "dying" or "dead," but later in the call stated that they were barely breathing. She was also unable to stay consistent with the amount of attackers that she said were there. She mentioned to the operator that the knife was lying in the garage and that she had already touched it. Then she said, "God...I bet if we could have gotten the prints maybe...maybe." According to experts, this type of reaction was very unusual for a mother. Instead of following her maternal instincts to save her children, Darlie appeared to be building an alibi and seeming to persuade the operator that it was not she who had committed the attack.

When police officers arrived, they found Darlie with serious looking yet superficial wounds. There were several cuts and scratches as well as a non-life threatening gash near the jugular vein of her neck. One of the officers instructed Darlie to get some towels so that pressure may be applied to her son's wounds, but she ignored him. The officer thought this was very strange even in the panicked state she displayed. She continued to scream that the intruder might still be in the garage. Paramedics arrived but soon realized that there was nothing they could do for the two boys that were already deceased or dying. Darlie continued to hold the bloody rag to her throat as the paramedics called for backup.

It was apparent that Devon had already died from his injuries, and his brother Damon was barely alive. Paramedics discovered two very large gashes in each of the boys' chests, most likely from a knife being thrust into them. The knife was driven so far down into the boys' chests that it penetrated into the concrete floor beneath the carpet. An IV was given to Damon in hopes that it would sustain him until they reached the hospital. It was undeniable that he was suffering the same fate as his brother. Damon was placed on the stretcher and into the ambulance. All life-saving maneuvers were attempted on him but with no success. He succumbed to his injuries on the way to Baylor Medical Center, which was just across town.

The police began the search throughout the house. They checked every room upstairs and downstairs. While upstairs, officers discovered a third child, an infant. He was lying in his crib crying, but showed no signs of bruising or any other type of trauma. Darin met them in the hallway and explained that this was the couple's youngest child, Drake.

The police then checked to see the state of the kitchen. This was the direction in which the killer was said to have fled. The floor was splattered with blood, the countertops blood smeared, the vacuum cleaner was knocked over, and a bloody butcher knife was lying on the kitchen countertop next to a woman's purse. Next to the purse was a set of expensive jewelry, which had been left untouched. The kitchen sink was spotless, as if it had recently been cleaned.

As the Routier home was being combed over by a large team of investigators, Darlie sat on the front porch while paramedics began working on her. They placed an IV in her arm and steri-strips across the cut on her neck. They escorted her to the ambulance, and they explained to Darin that she would need further treatment at Baylor Medical Center. Her husband said he would follow the ambulance, but, too shaken to drive, he requested that a neighbor, Tom Neal, drive him. Neal's wife stayed behind to look after the Routier's youngest child, Drake.

When Darlie arrived at the hospital, she was examined thoroughly. She underwent emergency surgery to repair her cuts. Her wounds looked to be serious, but in comparison to her sons' deep, violent, and fatal injuries, Darlie's were in fact superficial.

On the morning of June 14, 1996, the bodies of Devon, age six, and Damon, age five, were laid to rest in Rest Haven Memorial Park. The pastor began with a forty-five-minute sermon over the grave. A television crew was recording the funeral. However, they, as well as the Routiers, were unaware that investigators had also hidden their own cameras and microphones nearby. Television viewers were shocked when footage after the funeral showed Darlie laughing, chewing bubble gum, and spraying silly string over the freshly packed grave. She began singing "Happy Birthday" to her son Devon, whose birthday was being celebrated posthumously.

Within just eleven days of the murders, Darlie Routier was arrested. She was charged with capital murder in the death of her two sons. The coroner's conclusion was that the boys' wounds were so unbelievably savage, and Darlie's were described as "hesitation wounds" and possibly self-inflicted.

The Trial

On January 6, 1997, the capital murder trial of Darlie Routier began. The prosecution opened with the state's theory of the crime. According to the state prosecutors, Darlie was a woman that lived an extravagant lifestyle and the idea of motherhood threatened her ability to achieve this. They claimed that with her two sons dead, she could collect their life insurance policies and resume her wild spending ways. The prosecution also suggested that Darlie's behavior at Devon's graveside "birthday party" was not that of a grieving mother.

It was brought to the attention of the jury that Darlie never once asked about the condition of her sons when she was in the ambulance. The nurses at the hospital testified that Darlie never exhibited the traits of a grieving mother. They said she was more concerned about the fact that her prints were on the knife because she had picked it up at one point. Evidence from the crime scene was also presented to the jury. It was mentioned that blood and

Darlie's footprints were found underneath the vacuum cleaner. This would indicate that the vacuum was placed there after the crimes were committed. The only prints found were those of Darlie and her two sons. The blood on her nightshirt was that of her sons as well. Forensics suggested that it could have been sprayed when her arms were up in a stabbing motion.

An FBI special agent testified that if there had been an intruder, the window screen would not have been cut as it was found; an intruder would have merely removed it. Darlie's expensive jewelry that was still on the kitchen countertop dismissed the theory that this was a robbery. As far as the intruder being a rapist, the children would have most likely been used as leverage to get Darlie to submit, and they would have not been killed. In the FBI agent's opinion, the violent nature of the boys' wounds suggested that this was done out of extreme anger and was not committed by a stranger.

Darlie's defense attorney, Richard Mosty, gave his opening statements attempting to prove that she was not the crazed murderer that the prosecution had made her out to be. By this time, the defense knew that this was going to be a difficult task. Darlie's husband, Darin, was present in the witness box. He admitted to the family's financial problems, and he continued to attest to the fact that his wife was devastated by the death of their sons.

The biggest impact that the prosecution had was the opinion that the stab wounds on Darlie were "hesitation" wounds. However, the defense's forensic witness tried to lay doubt that these wounds were self-inflicted, as the gash on her neck came within 2 millimeters of her carotid artery and there were visible bruises on her arms, which indicated defensive wounds.

The defense presented forensic psychologist Lisa Clayton, an expert on the homicidal mind. She had previously interviewed Darlie and believed she was suffering from amnesia brought on by the trauma. Dr. Clayton was convinced she was innocent.

The final witness for the defense was a surprise to all: Darlie Routier herself. This would end up being a devastating mistake for the defense's case. They had tried to talk their client out of testifying, but Darlie persisted. On the stand, her defense team reviewed Darlie's life. She explained excerpts from her personal diary and described in detail the silly string graveside service, as well as details of the night of the murders.

When the defense stepped aside, the prosecution began to condemn her. They did not accept amnesia or her alibi. They did not accept one word that Darlie Routier had spoken, and they were going to convince the jury to do so as well. They asked her why she told several police officers different stories and why her dog never barked when the intruder entered the house. They asked why the kitchen sink had been cleaned of blood. The prosecutor looked her in the face and asked why she had lied, lied, and lied, and then walked away from the stand, leaving Darlie Routier sobbing and broken.

On February 1, 1997, after hours of deliberation, the jury found Darlie guilty of murdering Damon. Prosecutors did not try her for the death of Devon; this would be held in reserve in the event she was acquitted in her first trial. After three days, the judge looked down on her and read the decided penalty: Darlie Routier was sentenced to death by lethal injection.

Conclusion

On February 3, 2000, an episode of *20/20* aired that was titled, "Her Flesh and Blood." This episode examined the Darlie Routier case and revealed that the photographs of the bruising of her arms may not have been shown to the jury. The transcripts were reviewed, and over 33,000 errors and omissions were discovered. One juror that was interviewed on the broadcast admitted that he was peer-pressured into the guilty vote. He had also admitted that he never saw the mentioned photographs of the bruises.

In July of 2001, Darlie's lawyers filed for an appeal. They claimed that she deserved a new trial because the judge didn't properly handle the defense's conflict of interest. This was regarding the only other suspect which was her husband, Darin.

In June of 2002, a fingerprint expert, Dr. Richard Jantz, indicated that one of the unidentified fingerprints at the crime scene was indeed that of an adult, not a child.

This would support Darlie's claim that there was an intruder in the house the night of the murders. The defense argued that the prosecution should also turn over a specific piece of evidence for forensic testing: Darlie's nightgown that she was wearing at the time of the murders.

In 2011, Darin Routier filed for divorce from Darlie, having stayed married throughout the duration of the trial and her incarceration. He still claims his former wife is innocent. Darin and Darlie's youngest son, Drake, lives in Lubbock, Texas with his father.

As of 2014, Darlie Routier continues on death row waiting for lethal injection. She is being held in the Mountain View Unit, just outside of Gatesville, Texas. Petitions continue to be written in her defense, but are repeatedly delayed to lack of funding for DNA testing.

Darlie Routier has steadfastly maintained that she had nothing to do with the murders of her children.

A Poem by Darlie Routier

The following is a poem written by Darlie Routier to her sons nearly a year after the murders.

"Mommy We Love You"

"A double rainbow was seen over our home on 6-18-1996, the most beautiful rainbow I've ever seen." – Darlie Routier

I thought of you today, as I always do.
I thought of your smile and your laughter, too.
Your little hand pressed gently in mine,
no hurry or rush, no pressing of time.

I thought I would hold you forever,
but God took you home
to his kingdom in heaven.

There are so many words I never got to say,
so many games and silly things
we never got to play.
I saw the rainbow, not just one, but two
I knew it was a gift from your

brother and you.
My heart longs for you and I cry out in pain,
nothing in my life will ever be the same.
Come to me babies in my dream so true.
I need to hear your magic words,
"Mommy we love you."

In memory of my beautiful sons,
Devon and Damon.
By Darlie Routier
3-22-1997

Chapter 3: Susan Eubanks

Background

Susan Dianne Eubanks was born on June 26, 1964 and lived a troubled life. After the death of her mother when she was a young girl, she went on to marry John Armstrong and they had a boy named Brandon on July 13, 1983. Susan and John eventually divorced and she later married Eric Dale Eubanks, a cabinet-maker and Pop Warner football coach. Together they had three more children, Austin, Brigham, and Matthew. However, after nine years of marriage, Susan again wanted a divorce. There were several reasons for requesting the divorce that she cited before the judge. She stated that her husband beat her, often showcased erratic behavior, and had physically threatened her numerous times over the course of their marriage.

Ultimately, Susan stated she had become scared for her life because she was worried that her husband might cause her permanent harm. It is on record that she pleaded before the judge to issue a restraining order so that Eric Eubanks could be kept away from her as well as her children.

Like any other mother who recently breaks off her marriage, an instant burden of numerous financial responsibilities fell upon her shoulders. For Susan, the biggest burden of them all was to clear her credit card debts, which amounted to around $40,000. In addition to this, a separate court had given an explicit order to Susan to make a monthly payment of $341 in order to support Brandon, her son from her first marriage. It is easy to see that things were not really going very well for Susan Eubanks.

Once the divorce to Eubanks was finalized, Susan became involved with another man by the name of Rene Dobson, a construction worker. At this time, she was living in a ramshackle house with her four children in San Marcos, California. The plot of land on which her humble, two-bedroom house was situated was overrun with horses, chickens, and dogs.

The Murders

On October 27, 1997, Susan asked her eldest son, Brandon (then aged fourteen), to take care of the younger children while she and Dobson left to spend the day at a bar, drinking and watching a football game. The day quickly began to take a turn for the worse as the couple got in to a scuffle and a fight ensued.

They left the bar and headed for home. Once they reached home, Eubanks, according to Dobson, went "berserk." According to court documents, not only did she slash the tires of his car, she also broke his windshield and threw sugar in the gas tank. Then she trapped Dobson in the house and would not let him leave. He finally managed to escape via an open window and placed a call to the police station from a gas station located nearby. The police, upon arrival, escorted Dobson into the home so that he could take his possessions.

As per court documents, Dobson was placing his belongings in the trunk of his car when Susan came running out the door, shouting that she had been screwed by men her whole life, and that she had been beaten and raped. Dobson removed his belongings from the house and left. The police followed soon after.

All of this was happening before the eyes of Brandon Armstrong, Susan's eldest son. Seeing this, he ran to the nearest payphone as fast as he could, and called up Kathy Goohs, the mother of his best friend and the only person he thought he could rely on. Brandon asked Goohs to come to get him and the boys because he did not want the young children to witness the fight. Soon after, it is stated that Susan Eubanks herself called Goohs, and pleaded with her to take the children.

Goohs later revealed in court testimony that she never actually went to pick up the boys. She stated that because she did not have enough seat belts in the car, she was scared that the police might reprimand her when she arrived. Susan then called up John Armstrong, Brandon's father and her husband from the first marriage. John was living in Texas during this time. She told John that police had been over and investigations were underway over the scuffle that had taken place with Dobson, and that she had a strong fear that child protection services might come over and take away her children. Then, in a very disturbing move, Susan called up Eric Eubanks, the father of Matthew, Austin, and Brigham. The only message she left for him was, "Say goodbye." When Eric heard the message, he was obviously concerned for the safety of his children, and he called 911 to request a cursory check at the house to ensure the safety and well being of his children. It was this phone call that brought this heinous crime into the public eye.

When police arrived several hours later, they found a horrible scene. The sheriff, a hardened man who had seen a lot of violence over the years, later stated that in all his years, he had "never seen anything like it."

Upon arrival, the deputies forced their way in to the house and first inspected the master bedroom. There lying on the floor was Susan Eubanks with a towel clutched to the side of her abdomen. A revolver lay near her side, and when police removed the towel, they saw what appeared to be a gunshot wound that had, in all likelihood, been inflicted by Susan herself. Authorities immediately proceeded to check the other areas of the house, and found a horrific scene. Three of the boys, Austin (age seven), Matthew (age four), and Brigham (age six) were found in the bedroom. All of them had been shot at close range in the heads, leaving no chance of survival. Austin was found on the top bunk bed, while the other two boys lay dead on the lower bunk bed. Even though Austin and Brigham were dead, Matthew was still breathing. Matthew was rushed via helicopter to the Children's Hospital in San Diego, where he lost the battle of his life. He died at 4:30 p.m., only a short while after being brought to the hospital.

In the living room, police also found the body of fourteen-year-old Brandon. Brandon had also been shot in the head, and the police detected no pulse. He was declared dead on the spot.

A fifth child was also found in the home, the nephew of Susan Eubanks. He was five years old at the time, and was found virtually unharmed, though mentally scarred for life. According to court documents, the police found him in bed with the covers pulled up to his chin. The murders left the entire community in a state of shock and disbelief.

Susan Eubanks was taken to the Palomar Hospital, where she had to undergo an emergency surgical procedure. She was found with a significant loss of blood and was kept in the Intensive Care Unit. Eventually, however, she recovered.

Rod Englert, who later testified as the crime scene reconstructionist during the trials, stated that according to the scenario, the first one to be shot was Brandon. He stated that Brandon had likely been sitting on the floor of the living room when he had been hit with a shot straight to his left temple. As life left his body, Brandon slid to the floor in a slumping position, and that is when Susan shot Brandon again, this time in the neck. Englert also stated that Austin Eubanks, who was seated at the top bunk on the bed, had been shot in his left eye and he had his knees raised close to his face in a defensive position. The police also found two apparent misses, as bullet holes were present in the wall near the lower bunk bed, where Matthew and Brigham were shot.

At this point, all of the five bullets that are found in a standard .38 five shot revolver had been spent. After this, Susan opened the cylinder of the revolver, took out the used shell casings, and threw them in the bin. She then reloaded the gun and shot Brigham. Matthew Eubanks was the last person to die, as was revealed by Englert.

The Trial and Sentencing

Five days after the murders, Susan Dianne Eubanks was charged with four counts of first-degree murder and proceedings were initiated against her. The trial began in August 1999 and the prosecution stated that she had killed her four children in a fit of rage. They cited her previous scuffles with her boyfriends and ex-husbands (who had left her) as the reason for her rage. The prosecution stated that she wanted revenge.

As per the information revealed in court documents, five suicide notes were also discovered within the Eubanks household. One was addressed to Eric Eubanks, in which she stated, "you had betrayed me...I've lost everyone I ever loved. Now, it's time for you to do the same." Another letter was addressed to Rene Dobson. In this, Eubanks wrote, "you're the biggest liar to date. See ya. Ha. Ha." The third letter was written to John Armstrong, the father of Brandon. It read: "I know you'll hate me forever, but I can't let Brandon live without his brothers, so I did what I did." She also mentioned that she had been "strong for a long time," and was "tired of the hurt and the fights." Then, she wrote another letter to her sister and one to her niece, apologizing for her actions and asked that Matthew, the youngest, be buried with her only.

The defense lawyers argued that the murders were a result of her blacking out. They stated that because of her unstable mental condition, Susan did not really understand what she was doing. The defense lawyers argued that domestic disturbances, excessive drinking, and intake of prescription drugs had caused Susan to lose all feelings of emotion. The prosecutors countered this by stating that in order to complete the killings, she had to load her weapon twice, which gave her enough time to stop and reflect on what she was doing. Because she continued murdering after that pause, it showed that she was not suffering from a blackout at all. The attorneys also noted that she shot herself in order to get the charges reduced or to blame somebody else for the murder.

Court documents revealed that fifty bottles of prescription medications had been found in the Eubanks residence. This showed that Susan had been abusing prescription medications that had been prescribed to her after an injury she sustained on a job that required surgery.

After just two hours, the jury found Susan Dianne Eubanks to be guilty on all four counts of murder. As the penalty phase of her trial was underway, numerous relatives of John Armstrong testified about the impact that Brandon's death had on their own lives. Brandon's grandfather also gave a testimony, revealing two instances in which Susan had abused Brandon. Even her own sister, Linda Smith, recalled an incident in which Susan had revealed to her that she had rubbed the face of her nephew in a dirty diaper when she found out that the child had hid the diaper under the bed.

In return, the defense brought out evidence that the family had a history of alcoholism. Both the mother and father of Susan Eubanks were alcoholics, and Eubanks stated that when she was a young child, she had been beaten badly and abused by her mother, who used to drag her around by her hair. The defense argued that both of her parents had been caught having illicit affairs and her mother had died in a house fire when Susan was just eight years old. Without a mother figure in her life, Susan had to keep changing homes throughout the family, including living with an aunt who she claimed had abused her.

Certain relatives and friends of Susan also spoke up for her, stating that she was a very kind and loving mother and used to take good care of her children. They stated that Eubanks had experienced a very troublesome childhood in which she had been tortured for long periods of time, and made requests before the jury to not impose a death penalty sentence. As per court documents, Eric Eubanks reflected on their marriage, and stated that he still had some "loving feelings" toward his ex-wife. A correctional consultant was also brought into court, and he stated that Susan would not really be a danger to society if she were sentenced for life without the possibility of parole.

The court also concluded that throughout the trial, there were very minuscule legal errors, but none that could actually change the decision of the jury. It was also noted that before the murders had taken place, Susan had been threatening the men in her life that she would take revenge with them. The fact that she had shot herself in the stomach, while the other boys had all been shot in the head (hence effectively removing all chances of survival) was also brought up, and the prosecution stated that the primary purpose for this was that she thought the sentence could be reduced if she had inflicted harm on herself as well.

After two days, the jury returned with the verdict. To nobody's surprise, Susan Dianne Eubanks was sentenced to death. In October of 1999, the judge agreed with the jury's verdict. Susan Eubanks was then transferred to the Central California's Women's Facility, where she is currently on death row, awaiting her death. In 2011, she failed to win a reprieve from the Supreme Court of California, as the court upheld her death sentence.

Justice Ming W. Chin gave the ruling, rejecting her automatic appeal. At present, Susan Eubanks currently awaits the application of her death sentence, and constantly undergoes the torture of not knowing when a knock on her door might lead to her eventual death. As for the young children she brutally murdered in a fit of revenge, they are buried in graves in San Marcos. The community gave money for the headstones, primarily because the father of the children, Eric Dale Eubanks, was too distraught to make any sort of arrangements. Susan Eubanks not only put motherhood as a whole to shame, she also disgraced the blessings bestowed upon her by killing her four children in a brutal fit of rage. The community still grieves their deaths, and her actions serve as a stark reminder to the depths a person can fall to if they give in to their addictions.

Chapter 4: Lianne Smith

Background

Originally from Lichfield, Staffordshire, forty-five-year-old Lianne Smith was a mother of two, living with her long-term partner, Martin Smith. She had met Martin Smith through a dating agency back in 1992 in North Tyneside. At that period of time, Lianne was going through a divorce of her own. Together, the two began living in a small caravan that they had in Northumberland with her daughter and son from a previous marriage. They moved to Cumbria, where ironically, Lianne got a job as a child protection manager in the children's services department of the country's council. Before Martin Smith had gotten a job as a TV psychic, he was a singer in a band and performed in numerous clubs.

For more than a decade, the couple lived happily and had a daughter of their own, Rebecca. However, things really began to take a turn for the worse when Martin Smith was arrested in 2007 for allegations of sexually abusing his stepdaughter, Sarah. It was later revealed that Martin Smith had in fact, been sexually abusing his stepdaughter for over ten years. Sarah Richardson made a public statement in which she stated that he would try to hypnotize her by using ruses that she was going to fall asleep and would count down from ten. Even though she wouldn't actually fall asleep, she would continue to play along with his ruse because she knew he was going to subject her to sexual abuse regardless of whether she protested or not.

As news began to grow of Martin Smith's alleged rape and pedophilia, he was arrested by the police and questioned about the incidents. Before he could face charges, Martin and Lianne fled the country in 2007 and moved to Barcelona, Spain. However, back in the United Kingdom, the police weren't ready to give up on their search for Martin Smith. As a part of the thriving expatriate community of Spain, it wasn't difficult for Martin and Lianne to blend in, and soon, they were able to start a business together. At the time they had fled the country, their daughter, Rebecca, was three years of age. Their son, Daniel, was born in Spain in 2009. It was later revealed in court that there were still doubts over who the real father of Daniel and Rebecca was.

The police, on the other hand, had started a full-scale manhunt in order to track down Smith, and eventually did locate him in Barcelona. He was arrested and held in a Spanish prison in March 2010. He was then extradited back to the United Kingdom to appear before a court for the sex abuse charges that were levied against him. Throughout this time period, Lianne's mind was playing games with her. She feared for the life of her children, and was terrified that the British social services had arrived in Spain to take her children away from her. Her fear and confusion led her to make the only plausible choice that she thought she could make: she left the house with her two children and checked into a hotel one weekend. This would be the last weekend for young Daniel and Rebecca.

All evidence and court documents point to the fact that Lianne had planned out the murders of her two children before taking their lives. Soon after Martin was extradited back to the UK, Lianne took the children and checked in to the Costa Brava Resort in the Miramar Hotel, Lloret De Mar. As per the information revealed in the court documents, Lianne stated that she had given the kids a "perfect weekend" before killing them both.

Just before she murdered her children, she had created a very beautiful photo album, comprising of pictures of the "last wonderful holiday" that she had spent with her kids at Costa Brava. She also wrote a chilling farewell letter, and along with the album, had sent them to a publicist in the UK. She stated in the letter that she had managed to get out of the city before "they" took her children away from her, and that she had enclosed pictures of the last wonderful holiday she had spent with her kids, before the "events you will begin to hear about in the Press."

The next day, as the children were sleeping in their beds, she pinned down their legs with her own legs. This allowed her to prevent the children from moving so that she could place a plastic bag on the head of each child. The coroner's ruling was death by asphyxiation, as the kids died due to the lack of oxygen. At the time of their deaths, Rebecca was just five years old, while Daniel was only eleven months. Later on, Lianne Smith gave an interview in which she revealed the exact way by which she had killed her own children.

Surprisingly, she didn't call the police there and then. Instead, she waited a full day with her dead children in the same room with her. She tried to commit suicide but even though she had no problem taking the innocent lives of her two children, she couldn't bring herself to do it. After spending an entire day in the room with the deceased children, she called up the reception desk and asked them to call the police for her. Once the police arrived and found the two dead bodies, Lianne was immediately taken into custody. A video was made of the calm confession that

Smith gave to the detectives as she took a seat in the hotel room next to the one in which she had committed the murders and effortlessly explained her crimes. In the video, she claimed that she ended the lives of her two children after giving them the perfect weekend holiday. She also stated that she knew that the British social services were going to take her children away from her.

She claimed that she intended to die with the children, but couldn't do it. There was no need to hire a crime scene reconstructionist, as everything was explained by Lianne in chilling, explicit details. She revealed how she had killed young Daniel first. She stated how she had put a plastic bag on his head and asphyxiated him. She also stated that she knew when he was dead because she was the one holding the baby. The detectives asked her whether Rebecca had put up a struggle, to which she simply nodded.

After that, Lianne said she had spent the night cuddling her dead children in the hotel room, and wrote a number of notes. She wrote one to each of her dead children, stating that she was very sorry and that she had wanted to give them a "lovely life" together. After she was arrested, Lianne Smith was transferred to the Girona Prison and was treated by psychiatrist Dr. Harry Barker.

Spanish Police later revealed that Lianne Smith had suffocated her two children in Room 101 of the Hotel Miramar. During their time in prison, both Martin and Lianne wrote each other frequently. A source at the prison where Lianne was being held revealed that Lianne believed that Martin was innocent, and she was devoted to him. The source also stated that the letters that she received and wrote were considered to be very important to her. Every month, Martin was allowed to make an eight-minute phone call to Lianne, and she had told all of the people in prison that this was the reason why she was still living. She told several people at the prison that if Martin wasn't alive, she would have killed herself long ago to be with her children. At one point she revealed to a psychiatrist that she had killed her children "out of love."

Even though she admits to smothering the children, she denies murdering them, stating that she was mentally ill at the time.

The Trial

The trial of Lianne Smith was not a very long one, as one might expect. Her case was heard at the Provincial Court in Girona, and it was decided that she was criminally responsible for the murder of her two children. The jury was shown the chilling video that had been shot when the police had arrived on the scene, in which she explained to the detectives how she had killed her children.

The prosecution had argued for the maximum sentence of 34 years, however she received 15 years for the murder of each child, making it a total of 30 years without parole. Judge Adolfo Garcia Morales, who presided over the case, revealed in a public statement sent to the media how the killings had taken place and why he was imposing the minimum sentence for the murders committed by Lianne Smith because he believed that she was suffering from a mental disturbance when she committed the crimes.

He started by saying that the sleeping

children were virtually incapable of defending themselves in any possible way, and that it was obvious that Lianne had planned the whole thing all along. The defense claimed that she was mentally insane and should not be tried for the maximum sentence. However, the jurors rejected this claim, as it was obvious that she had premeditated the whole scenario before committing the murders.

The court was told how Lianne Smith was "pathologically obsessed" with her long time partner, Martin Smith. Even though Lianne tried to plead her mentally disturbed state, all appeals were waived and she was convicted. In the statement given by Judge Adolfo, the jury had stressed that the mental disturbance suffered by Smith was not as important as the defense made it out to be. He also claimed that the jurors had come to this conclusion after a number of incidents. He stated that the numerous suicide attempts made by Smith played a major role, as well as the fact that in the statement she gave to the police, she appeared completely calm and normal and hadn't made any mistakes at all when describing what had actually transpired. The evidence put forth was also of vital use, as it included numerous coherent notes made by Smith, including that she even calculated the amount of money that she owed the hotel.

Unfortunately for her, the misery was far from over. Stunning revelations came to the forefront that Lianne Smith had once engaged in prostitution, and catered to clients all over the North of England. It was stated that Martin Smith would drive her to the houses of clients and would then wait out in the car. This mystery was further deepened by the fact that Rebecca was born in Blackpool, Lancashire in 2004, while Daniel was born in Barcelona in 2009. These revelations have never been confirmed nor denied by the family of Lianne Smith.

Even though it was mentioned in the trial that Martin Smith fathered the children, this claim was put in doubt when Interpol revealed that the DNA sample that was sent by the prosecution might not have belonged to Martin Smith at all. Rebecca's birth certificate stated her father was Martin Anthony Smith, however, this was also the period of time when Martin and Lianne had called off the relationship for five months. Daniel was conceived in 2008 when Martin was forty-two years old, in Barcelona, the court heard. However, no formal documents as to the birth of the child could be produced.

The jury consisted of two women and seven men, and just after eight hours of deliberation, the verdict was revealed that the jury believed Lianne Smith to be "fully conscious" at the time of the murders, and that she knew what she was doing as she smothered both Daniel and Rebecca. As the unanimous guilty verdict was announced in Court, Lianne Smith just stared blankly at the floor, devoid of emotion.

After the verdict was revealed, Lianne's twenty-one-year-old son, Chris Smith, revealed that he was absolutely disgusted at the "abominable" murders that his mother had committed. Chris stated that the verdict brought an end to his "worst nightmare." Talking to *The Daily Mirror*, Chris stated that he had really wanted to be there to see the emotions of guilt that his mother might have felt when the word 'guilty' had been announced. He stated that it was impossible to forgive her. Lianne's eldest daughter, Sarah Richardson, also stated that she was never going to forgive her mother.

In her defense, Lianne stated that she felt she had been pushed in to a corner, and that she had always intended to go with her children, together. Instead of serving her sentence in a psychiatric hospital, Lianne will be serving her 30 years in a standard prison somewhere in Catalonia. Even after being sentenced to prison, things didn't change for Lianne. As revealed by guards and inmates where she is currently serving her sentence, Lianne's only source of hope to live was Martin. In January 2012, Martin Smith was found dead in his cell after he committed suicide.

A spokesman for the Prison Service revealed that Martin Smith had committed suicide after eating his evening meal. He was forty-six years old and hanged himself at the HMP Manchester. The news was revealed to Lianne Smith by a team consisting of a psychiatrist, a social worker, and an official of the British Embassy. As soon as the news was revealed to her, she was taken from the standard hospital ward at the prison where she was being held under low-level observation to a secure complex in the jail that is focused on psychiatry, and put on twenty-four-hour surveillance under the observation of a team of specialists. Now, Lianne serves her time under the constant surveillance of the suicide watch, biding her days without any reprieve.

Fathers

The first four Filicide cases have been on mothers. There has been no shortage of fathers that have committed filicide either. Before we continue, here is a short prologue about fathers and history that I think you will find interesting.

No matter how you look at it, killing somebody is a heinous, unforgivable thing. All religions condemn it, all teachings go against it, and yet man has killed billions over the ages. We are so fond of killing that the desire practically runs inside us. Some people kill for fun, even though they could be caught, jailed, and prosecuted. Others kill out of revenge. The same fate befalls them. However, there are those who kill for no apparent reason and who blame their mental conditions for these killings. They do not accept that whatever happened was thought by their mind and implemented by their body.

Nowadays, you hear about killing a lot. In every country, the average death toll of people who are killed on a daily basis is rising. As expected, most of these deaths are borne out of personal enmity. For the investigators and the police, it is much easier to come to a rational conclusion about the motive of such deaths because it is so evidently clear. Connecting the dots is easy because most murderers aren't exactly silent assassins or professionals.

However, every so often, there comes along a case that is virtually impossible to explain. It becomes impossible to truly understand what exactly led to the killings, and even if the killer confesses, he or she fails to provide a good enough theory that might support his or her actions. For the third party, you and I, it becomes baffling. How do you explain the killing of children by their own father? Was he mentally handicapped? Even if he was mentally handicapped, how could he raise children, only to kill them with his own hands? These are just some of the answers that we crave, yet might never get. The mind of a man is truly a wonderful, yet extremely dangerous thing. It can lead him to do amazing things, or it can lead to massive destruction.

Count out all the great wars, the huge atrocities that have been committed, and then keep them aside. This is not about war. This is not about a mass murder. This is about a crime much greater than all of these combined. This story is about a father who chose to take the wrong path, and ended up murdering his own, beloved children. It truly makes one think about how low a person can fall if circumstances do not go according to his own way, and it really makes one think, *is this even possible?*

Well, if you believe in historical evidence, killing one's own children has been around for centuries. Men used to bury their daughters alive as soon as they were born, just because they wanted a son. In certain ages, tyrants who ruled the lands used to order all newborns to be buried immediately because they thought that these young babies would grow up and challenge them to the throne. But how do you explain the killing of grown children? I don't think anybody can give an explanation that will truly convince the human heart.

Chapter 5: Alan Bristol

Background

Alan and Christine Bristol of New Zealand had been together for quite a while. Christine, if you are wondering, was the wife of Alan Bristol. However, even before they married, Christine had been a victim to domestic violence at the hands of Alan. Before they had even been engaged, the two had been living together for around eighteen months. According to Christine, Alan began physically abusing her after they had been living together for about six months. In her own words, he used to "punch and throw me around." What started off as a love affair quickly turned into something much more dangerous.

According to Christine, Alan would beat her up almost every week, sometimes even several times in a week, and she often had a number of different bruises, as well as black eyes. She also revealed that Alan would use his physical presence to intimidate her, and more often than not, would belittle her any way that he could. Christine later revealed that Alan wanted to dominate any way he could and he would stop at nothing to get the upper hand; even resorting to using children to pressurize her.

Christine broke off her engagement with Alan in December of 1985. She went to court and also got an interim non-molestation order. However, it wasn't very long before she realized that she had become pregnant with the couple's first child, Tiffany. She later stated that she had "always wanted to do the right thing," and because of that, she decided to reconcile with Alan. She stated that Alan would keep a check on whom she was getting mail from and would constantly be asking questions about where she was going, what she was doing, etc.

When Tiffany was born, he tried to control his abuse. Unfortunately, he couldn't. Not only would he abuse her physically, he would mentally torture her as well, and then rape her. And, according to Christine, the next morning he would act as if nothing had happened; he would bring flowers and chocolates to show that he was not a bad person and did not mean to hurt her. According to Christine, Alan always knew where to hit her so that the bruises wouldn't show. He would also warn her that it was useless telling anybody about it, because he hailed from an important family, while she was a nobody. Yet, she continued to live with him.

Throughout the relationship, Christine left Alan several times, but he would always persuade her to come back. Alan was extremely jealous and possessive about Christine, and this made her feel like a "caged animal." Alan's constant physical torture was reported to the police over a dozen times. It was either Christine calling the police, or it was her brothers. However, as Christine later stated, she thought the police were never really interested, even though she showed them the strangle marks and the bruises.

Once, Alan was strangling her in their home on Puriri Street when the police arrived. Instead of arresting him, they asked Alan to take his things and leave rather than provoking the situation further. There were many times when Christine would separate from her husband and move away, and it was during one of these separation phases in 1989 when she had him arrested for being in an enclosed yard. Christine stated that he kept knocking on her windows and doors. During the same year, Christine also started to receive numerous calls from anonymous callers, and there was also an arson attack at her residence.

Christine later stated that even though Alan was quite violent towards her, he was actually a good father, but she was always frightened for the kids. Until 1993, the story of mental and physical abuse continued to persist. Then, Christine decided to make a change. She told him that the marriage was over, and throughout the next two days until she left the house, Alan beat her and shouted at her. At that time, her youngest kid was just 10 months old.

Over the years, Christine had gotten non-molestation and non-violence orders from the court several times. However, in

September 1993, the court issued a memorandum that placed her non-molestation order in limbo until the issue of the custody of the children was sorted out. As a result, the protection she had from Alan's intimidating behavior was waived off indefinitely. Things had begun heating up between the two by that point, and they were often getting back together and separating again and again. At this point in time, he was beating Christine in front of the children as well.

The Murders

The beatings had become a lot more frequent by that point in time. Even though they had been separated, Christine often used to visit with the kids when they were with Alan. Whenever Christine would go on an access visit, Alan would threaten and beat her. Once, she had filed an official complaint to the police, and he had been called in for questioning. When she visited the children on the next access visit, he threatened her with a knife against her throat. Eventually, she was able to talk him down and Christine was able to leave with the younger children.

Christine soon realized that it had become a big risk to be in the house alone with Alan when she went to pick up the children, so she would often take somebody along in the car with her. She did this even though Alan had explicitly asked her not to bring anybody or she would not get the children. Once, they had gotten into a scuffle and Alan had tried to rape her. To get herself away, Christine had used her force to twist his arm and escape.

Soon after, she began to fear that Alan would turn on the children. She later stated that he had often said things like, "If I can't have you, nobody will," and even though she had never paid much heed to his threats, she soon feared it might not be long before he started turning on the children.

Since Alan had interim custody of their three daughters on the weekend, Christine had to drop the children off each weekend. During one of those drop offs, they got in to a fight again and this time, Alan took her car keys, tore off her under garments and shoved the keys in her crotch, all while the three young daughters stared at what was happening. After this particular incident, Christine filed charges and applied for sole custody of her daughters.

That same night, Alan told his mother that if Christine made her charges stick, he would be jailed for 10 years. If she was able to get the indecent assault charge levied on him, he would be jailed for twenty years. He then stated the worst thing about the entire situation was that she was going for the children.

On February 2, 1994, the fear of conviction and losing custody of his children drove him to put the three girls in the backseat of his hatchback car, which was parked in the driveway. At that time, Alan was living in a remote home. He then took out the swimming pool hose and connected one end to the exhaust and the other end to the front windows of the car. Then he turned on the ignition. The next day, George Bristol, Alan's father, discovered the car and the lifeless bodies of Alan, and his three daughters Tiffany (aged seven), Holly (aged three), and Claudia (just eighteen months). By this period of time, the separation between Alan and Christine had been in effect for eight months.

Alan Bristol and his daughters were kept in the morgue, where Christine would visit them everyday. Later on, she stated that she would only visit because she wanted to see him "cold." The investigations carried out by the police revealed that Alan Bristol had left no notes that provided an insight as to why he had carried out his actions. Police investigations also revealed that the children never even realized what was happening. As per the crime scene experts, the children were dead within three minutes, tops.

However, Alan did not die with the children. Upon realizing what he had done as well as the consequences of his actions, Alan had turned off the ignition. According to the crime scene experts, it took Alan about fifteen minutes to die, but unlike the children, Alan actually struggled. When he was found, it appeared as if he had just turned the ignition off. The investigators concluded that everything had been set up beforehand, primarily due to the usage of the swimming pool hose. When Christine was asked why he would do such a thing, her only reply was that he wanted to get back at her. She believed that Alan had realized that he was going to be exposed before the world as to the kind of person he was, and this did not sit well with him. More importantly, it was obvious that he was going to lose custody of the children.

The Aftermath

Because Alan Bristol had killed himself along with his three children, there were no trials, since there was nothing to really fight for. However, a report was compiled that provided an insight into the death of the children, which revealed a number of interesting things. First of all, it revealed that the courts had never received an opportunity to listen to the parties that were providing evidence, or to even test the truth of the allegations that were made. The final conclusion given in the report was that the court had nothing before it that could have allowed it to entertain the possibility that Alan Bristol might act the way he did.

However, during that same period of time, the overall number of incidents related to domestic violence had increased considerably in New Zealand. As a result, Sir Ronald Davison, the now retired Chief Justice, filed a report questioning whether it was time to implement statutory intervention to help women who had been physically and mentally harmed by their husbands, as well as children. The report highlighted a model that was growing rapidly in those times, now known as the power and control model. This model generally pertains to the use of domestic violence by men against women in order to assert their dominance and control.

The report also made numerous recommendations. First and foremost, it called on the courts to levy stricter penalties for any breaches in non-violence orders. Then, it also asked for the courts to be fully satisfied as to whether the allegations regarding domestic violence were true or not before it decided to pass consent orders. The report also provided a recommendation in which it stated that violent parents should be restricted from gaining access to their children.

After this report was filed, an amendment was made in the Guardianship Act. A new addition was made in the form of subsection 16A, B, and C in late 1995. Section 16B provided a presumption that in any case where a parent was found to be a violent person, any access to the child, or any sort of contact, would be done under the supervision until the Court was fully satisfied that the child was safe in the hands of that violent parent.

During the same time period, the Domestic Violence Act was also put in effect. The Domestic Violence Act gave a clear depiction of violence, stating that it includes physiological, sexual, and physical violence. The previous orders, named the non-molestation order and the non-violence order were both replaced by one distinct order, known as the protection order. The protection order clearly restricts the violent parent from meeting the victim or any child of the victim that might have been born when the two were in a relationship. The restriction could, however, be waived off by the victim in order to allow the violent party to meet with her.

Christine Bristol was obviously distraught after the ordeal, and she continued to blame the courts for not taking proper action against Alan when things could have been stopped from getting out of hand. When asked about what she thought could have been done by the legal system in order to improve her situation, she stated that over the passage of time, she had become extremely tired of all that was happening. As a result, she often thought about letting Tiffany be with Alan. She has often stated on record that she wanted complete protection from Alan. She also stated that her solicitor had not told her about her rights: what she could do and could not do. She stated that throughout the time that she was moving in and out of courts, she didn't even have an idea about what her basic rights were. She also stated that she didn't even know whether any support groups existed to help her out. She believed that Alan knew where he was going, and that he had an idea of the legal system as well as the exploits that he could use against her.

The death of Claudia, Holly, and Tiffany proved to be a major source of reform in the legislature in New Zealand. A number of new bills were passed, and the government made numerous editions to the existing legislature that pertains to domestic violence as well as the clear definition of violence itself. After the deaths of her children, Christine Bristol was shell shocked, obviously. She has stated that it is very difficult for her to view layers of any kind, especially in wedding cakes, because they remind her of the way that her children were laid out to rest in their final resting places.

When the children's bodies were in the morgue, Christine studied the bruises on their bodies. She also brought family clothes that the girls had liked to the morgue and adorned them in these clothes, as a form of a final goodbye. She now spends her time reviewing changes in the government legislature and working with NGOs in order to make sure that other instances of child and partner abuse are minimized as much as possible. Christine currently resides in her homeland with her family.

Chapter 6: Jeffrey MacDonald

Background

Jeffrey Robert MacDonald was born in Jamaica, Queens, in New York City in the year 1943. He was the second of three siblings, born to parents Robert and Dorothy MacDonald. He studied at the Patchogue High School, where he was deemed to have a very bright future. Jeffrey received the highest voting for the titles "most likely to succeed," as well as "most popular boy." During his high school years, Jeffrey won a scholarship to Princeton University. While he was at Princeton, Jeffrey became romantically involved with Colette Stevenson. He had previously been with Colette during high school, although they had not been involved romantically. While he was studying at Princeton, Colette was studying at Skidmore College. It was during those college years, on September 14, 1963, when Jeffrey learned that Colette was pregnant with his first child. As a result of this, Jeff decided to marry Colette. On April 18, 1964, Colette MacDonald gave birth to Kimberly, their first daughter.

Jeffrey studied at Princeton for three years, after which he decided to move with his family to Chicago in 1964. In Chicago, he got acceptance from the Northwestern University Medical School, and enrolled there. It was during this time when the couple gave birth to their second child, Kristen, on May 8, 1967. The next year, Jeffrey graduated from medical school and also managed to complete an internship based in New York City, at the Columbia Presbyterian Medical Center. After this, Jeffrey decided to join the army, a decision he went through with on July 1, 1969. Soon after, the family of four moved to live in Fort Bragg, North Carolina. Jeffrey MacDonald held the rank of Captain during his stint in the army. In September of 1969, Jeffrey got his first assignment: he was assigned as a Group Surgeon to the Green Berets to the 3rd Special Forces.

Colette was very happy with Jeffrey

and never had any problems. Unlike other unstable husbands, Jeffrey didn't beat her, use physical dominance, or ever got angry with her. In fact, just a few months prior to their deaths, Colette had written a Christmas card to some of her friends telling of the "all paid expense" that was given to them by the Army, and how she was so relaxed. She also wrote that they were expecting a son in July. Colette had always planned that once Jeffrey was done with his military duties, the couple and their children would move to a farm and raise five children and keep all kinds of pets, ranging from rabbits to horses.

Throughout his life, Jeffrey had been smart and successful. He was handsome and hardworking and intelligent. He had been the high school quarterback and the president of student council. There was nothing during his lifetime that could suggest that Jeffrey might turn out to be such a dangerous person. According to Colette, she was living the dream. She had a loving husband, two beautiful daughters and a son was on the way. Unfortunately, things changed very quickly for the couple and their two children, presumably because of a fit of rage.

The Murders

Their fairy tale love story skidded to a halt and turned in to a horror story on a cold and rainy morning. It was 3:42 a.m. on the morning of February 17, 1970 when an operator received a phone call in Fayetteville, North Carolina, from a man who referred to himself as Captain MacDonald. He was begging the operator to call the police as well as an ambulance to their home address, which was at 554 Castle Drive. In a very weak voice, he was only able to say the words "stabbing." The operator was obviously shocked at such a call, and in a panicked state, immediately patched the call to the headquarters of the military police in Ford Bragg. Captain MacDonald repeated his plea for help to the military police, who immediately sprung in to action.

The desk sergeant who took the call immediately sent several military police officers (MPs) to the address provided by Jeffrey MacDonald, but he was unable to get the base hospital to dispatch an ambulance to 554 Castle Drive until after the MPs had already stormed the household and decided whether the ambulance was actually required or not. As the MPs traveled to Jeffrey's household, one of them, Kenneth Mica, later reported that he saw a very weird sight just three blocks away from the house of Captain MacDonald. A young woman stood in a raincoat and a wide brimmed floppy hat, at 3:55 a.m. in the morning. She wasn't moving around, just standing. Kenneth later stated that if it wasn't a distress call from Captain MacDonald, he and his partner would have stopped their vehicles and inquired about the woman's whereabouts as well as what she was doing there.

Soon after, more than a dozen MPs showed up at 554 Castle Drive. The house was dark and the front door was locked. The MPs initially thought that they had been called in to settle a dispute regarding domestic disruption. The MPs knocked on the front door, but nobody answered. After a bit of waiting, they headed to the back of the house, where they saw that the screen door at the back was closed and unlocked and the back door was ajar. What they were about to see was horrifying.

As soon as they entered the master bedroom, they saw the body of Colette MacDonald. She was twenty-six years old at the time. She was lying on her back, with her legs spread and blood all over her. There were numerous injuries to her face and her head, as though somebody had clubbed her head in. A portion of her naked chest was exposed, while one of her breasts was covered partially by a blue pajama top that had been badly torn. Right next to her, with his head placed on her lifeless shoulder, was Captain MacDonald. Jeffrey wore nothing but blue pajama bottoms and when Kenneth Mica bent down beside him, MacDonald asked about his kids. He said he had heard them crying.

As soon as he heard this, Mica and the other MPs ran straight to the other rooms in search for the children. In one of the bedrooms, he found Kimberly, who was five years old at that time. She was in bed, tucked under the covers. However, as Kenneth aimed the flashlight over her body, the sight that followed sickened him to his stomach. Somebody had clubbed her head in, and she had been stabbed in the neck numerous times. Right across the hall, the MPs found the lifeless body of two-year-old

Kristen, who was lying on her bed, dead from the numerous stab wounds she had received in her chest and her back. Kenneth went back to Captain MacDonald and asked him who had done this to them, to which MacDonald replied that there were three men and a woman. One was black, wearing a field jacket and sergeant's stripes, while the woman had blond hair and wore a floppy hat. Kenneth Mica tried to relay this information to his Lieutenant, but he was busy writing out the details.

As the ambulance began to stretcher off Jeffrey MacDonald, Mica noted that he was concerned only for his kids. Colette had been clubbed repeatedly, both of her arms had been broken, and she had been stabbed a total of thirty-seven times: twenty-one times with an ice pick and sixteen times with a knife. Five-year-old Kimberly had been stabbed anywhere between five to eight times. The smallest of the lot, Kristen had been stabbed with a knife thirty-three times and fifteen times with an ice pick.

The Aftermath

Once Jeffrey was able to speak about the incident, he stated that he had been sleeping on the couch after watching some late night television when he heard his wife screaming. He then stated a black man tied him up and beat him until he was unconscious. He said there were also two white men and a woman who chanted, "kill the pigs, acid is groovy." When he awoke, he saw Colette lying dead beside him, and he tried to revive her with mouth-to-mouth CPR, but to no avail. Failing that, he called the ambulance.

In response to his story, the Army Criminal Investigation Command (CID) decided to send out a rookie, an inexperienced investigator by the name of William Ivory. After taking a look at the crime scene and analyzing the details, Ivory decided that MacDonald had created the whole story, and that MacDonald himself was the real killer. He managed to persuade those in his chain of command that MacDonald was the killer, and subsequently, the army put all of its efforts into convicting MacDonald. Even though there were several pieces of evidences available that there were others involved in the attack, the Army refused to analyze those pieces of evidence.

There were a number of bad decisions made on the part of the Army that followed afterwards. First of all, investigations were hampered severely because of the fiasco at the crime scene. Evidence had been touched by the MPs, to the point that one of the MPs had even picked up a dangling receiver and used it to call the ambulance. The ambulance driver had moved things around in the crime scene, which ultimately led William Ivory to believe that MacDonald was behind the attack. The same driver also stole MacDonald's wallet. The young woman in the floppy hat who was spotted near the house was later identified to be Helena Stoeckley, who was deeply into drugs and witchcraft. However, Ivory had failed to make any sort of connection.

According to the CID, the living room where Jeffrey said to have fought the assailants had not been disturbed much, and certainly showed no signs of a struggle. MacDonald claimed that his pajamas had been torn in the living room, but no fibers were found. Instead, fibers were found under the bodies of Colette, Kimberly, and Kristen. The CID came to the conclusion that the fight had started in the master bedroom between the husband and wife, possibly about Kristen's bed-wetting that night. Investigators said that it was likely that Colette hit Jeffrey with a hairbrush on the forehead, giving him the head wound. At that point, Jeffrey retaliated by using a piece of lumber to repeatedly club Colette. During this time, Kimberly might have walked in. Since her brain serum was found in the doorway, it is likely that she had been struck by accident at least once. Once MacDonald thought that Colette had died, he carried Kimberly, who had been wounded fatally, to her bedroom and stabbed her repeatedly. Then, he went to Kristen's room to kill off the last potential witness. At this point, it is likely that Colette intervened, but Jeffrey killed them both.

Then, as per the theory of the CID, MacDonald tried to cover the murders up by using a story from the articles about the Manson family that he had read in *Esquire* magazine. He took a scalpel and stabbed himself. This formal report was put before a judge, and on April 6, 1970, just a month and a half after the murders, Army investigators began interrogating MacDonald. On May 1, the Army placed formal charges on Jeffrey MacDonald for the brutal murder of his family.

***

Now, whenever a member of the armed forces is charged with a crime, Article 32 of the Uniform Code of Military Justice comes into effect. This article requires that a separate officer be appointed to analyze whether there is truth to these charges or not, as well as give recommendations on the next steps to be taken on the case. The officer, in this case, was Warren V. Rock. The lawyer selected for Jeffrey MacDonald was Bernard Segal. Bernard Segal focused primarily on the incompetence shown by the Army in compiling the evidence, stating numerous instances in which crime scene control was completely abolished, as well as the disruptions that were caused by the MPs during their movements in the household.

Bernard Segal came up with several

pieces of evidence that showcased the incompetence of the Army, especially in locating Helena Stoeckley, who was a known drug user and according to witnesses, had already claimed involvement in the crimes. As a result of this, on October 13, 1970, Colonel Rock issued the verdict that all charges against Captain Jeffrey MacDonald be dismissed, since they were untrue. He was given an honorable discharge from the Army, and returned back to New York.

***

After the hearing, Jeffrey started working as a doctor again. During this time, Jeffrey's father in law, Freddie Kassab, turned against him. Along with investigators of the U.S. Army, Kassab had investigated the crime scene for several hours before finally coming to the conclusion that MacDonald committed the crimes himself. He then filed a citizen's complaint. The case remained unopened for several years, until finally, on January 24, 1975, a grand jury in North Carolina indicted MacDonald after deliberating for just one hour. He was arrested in California. He was freed on bail on January

31, pending disposition of charges after posting a bail of $100,000.

The murder trial began on July 16, 1979 and finally, on August 29, 1979, MacDonald was convicted of one charge of first-degree murder as well as two charges of second-degree murder. He was ordered to serve three life terms. In an odd turn of events, MacDonald's conviction was reversed in 1980, but later that year, the Fourth Circuit Court ensured that the earlier decision stood. Judge Dupree rejected all defense motions for a new trial in 1985.

Until 1992, Dupree continued to deny several motions and petitions filed by the defense.

***

In 2002, MacDonald married his second wife, Kathryn Kurichh, a pen pal he met while serving his prison sentence. She owns a drama school for children in Maryland. Jeffrey is still incarcerated in California and takes classes for nutrition, heart health, and smoking cessation. A parole hearing was scheduled in 2005, where Jeffrey refused to admit guilt and stated that he was factually innocent. Immediately, the hearing was dismissed. The next parole hearing is now scheduled in the year 2020. To this day, it is unclear whether Jeffrey MacDonald actually killed his wife and children, but what actually happened was a brutal act that took the lives of three beautiful souls. Was Jeffrey MacDonald wrongfully imprisoned for killing his family? Many believe so. You be the judge on this case.

Most people spend their entire lives working away; earning a wage that is barely able to support them and their families, hardly being able to live in peace. However, there are others who get their break much quicker. They work hard in their early years, get a good education, and then strive to do even bigger and better things. Common sense states that these people are more mentally stable, because they have fewer worries. Even though this is a very vague statement, it is not entirely untrue. The most important thing to keep in mind here is that the human brain is an extremely unstable thing. It is capable of doing things we often think impossible. As is the case with everything in life, impossible is a word that can be used in two different ways: positive and negative.

In his rage, man is capable of doing the most heinous tasks. All of the great men have often reiterated the importance of controlling one's emotions when he is in a rage, because if let loose, these emotions can lead to actions that have potentially damaging repercussions. Decisions taken in anger seldom yield positive results, and more often than not, lead to further misery. That is why it is always stated to avoid letting your emotions get the best of you.

Anger, rage, and guilt are three such emotions that can drive a person to the point of madness. What is madness? What actions lead to a man being called "mad"? The dictionary says that any person who is carried away by intense anger can't be called mad. Anger is the state of mind when a person fails to think properly. He forgets whom he loves, what he cares for, and what he was tasked with. There is just one desire on his mind: to destroy. In his rage, man can destroy anything that is around him.

He can destroy relationships, the lives of his people, he can destroy homes, and most important of all, he can destroy love. All this can be destroyed in a jiffy if man makes some rash moves during his rage. Yet, we fail to learn from our mistakes, refusing to address this negligence. Most of us are slaves to our own habits, yet we never try to curb those habits. As a result of this, man is still struggling to reach his full potential.

They say that family is the closest thing, and yet the family suffers most if a person in rage takes out their anger on them. How could a person like Jeffrey MacDonald become so angry that he ends up killing his beloved children and his wife? We'll never be able to truly understand the circumstances that can lead the human mind into committing such heinous crimes against their loved ones. This is the story of Jeffrey MacDonald, who had everything going for him. He had a pretty wife, beautiful children, and a stable job, but he chose to throw it all away. Or someone did.

Chapter 7: Deanna Laney

Background

New Chappell Hill, Texas is a quiet town just seven miles south of Tyler, Texas. It is a town known to be a religious and well-established place to raise a family. This was the residence of Deanna Laney, her husband Keith, and their three sons, Joshua, Luke, and Aaron, ages eight, six, and fourteen months.

Deanna LaJune Boatright was born July 13, 1964, in East Texas. She attended Chapell Hill High School for her freshman, sophomore, and junior years, and she was a popular girl who was active in varsity volleyball and the Future Homemakers of America organization. She was heavily involved in extracurricular activities as well. For unknown reasons, Deanna moved to Tyler High School to complete her senior year.

Records indicate that Deanna was raised in a stable and devoutly Christian home. Her family attended church on a regular basis, which was the First Assembly of God where Deanna's brother-in-law was the pastor. According to friends and family, she had no signs of mental instability growing up, nor any indications of family problems. She appeared to be a very stable, happy, and intelligent girl.

Deanna and Keith Laney were married on October 13, 1984, just a few years after she graduated from Tyler High School. The couple always appeared happy and smiling and never showed any signs of marital trouble. Ten years went by before the Laneys had their first child. Joshua Keith Laney was born on July 28, 1994. This was just fifteen days after Deanna's thirtieth birthday. Their second son, Luke Allen Laney, was born two years later on September 9, 1996. Finally, on February 13, 2002, Aaron James Laney was born.

Deanna was a stay-at-home mom, as most mothers were in this rural area of Texas. She tended to the housework daily, cooked, and home-schooled the children while her husband was at work. Keith, an air compressor repairman, made a modest income, yet they somehow made ends meet. Deanna appeared to most of her acquaintances as a good mother as well as a devout Christian. She and her family attended church every chance they got. The couple followed a fundamentalist Christian belief that kept them mostly at home and didn't allow for much of a social life; some thought that the Laneys' religious beliefs were a bit extreme.

There were no signs of postpartum depression after the births of her children. However, after Aaron was born, Deanna started to feel a bit overwhelmed. Aaron was a very active child, and this became a distraction when Deanna tried to home-school the older children. Keith had suggested to her that they send Joshua and Luke to a public or private school the following year to relieve Deanna of the home-schooling responsibilities and alleviate some of the stress.

Eventually, Deanna's mental state began to take a downward turn. She started having delusions and, at times, seemed to step out of reality. On one occasion, her youngest son, Aaron, had difficulties with bowel movements. To Deanna, it was a sign that the child was not digesting the Word of God properly. She would have hallucinations that God was speaking to her and she believed God was giving her signs or messages. At times, she would claim that she smelled sulfur and that this was a sign the devil was near. She had one particular paranoid delusion that her family would leave a restaurant and be killed in a car crash. This delusion occurred while she was at home cooking dinner.

Deanna was a member of the choir, a youth sponsor, and she also attended church up to three times a week. The Laneys were considered very strong members and leaders of their church.

Deanna's deteriorating mental state became more apparent to her sister when she began to withdraw from most social situations. She began losing weight, stopped going out to dinner with the family, and no longer went shopping as she usually did. She began withdrawing from friends and family, but spoke quickly, fasted, and started reading the bible more often.

Deanna was showing signs of the impending tragedy that would occur just a few weeks later.

During the first week of May in 2003, Deanna began having even more severe hallucinations. One day, her youngest son, Aaron, was playing in his room. He was holding a toy spear in one hand and a frog by the neck in the other while rocking back and forth. Deanna believed this was a sign from God that she should kill her children by strangulation or stabbing to test her faith in Him. Aaron later took a small black horse out of the toy chest and began playing with it. To her, the black horse was a sign of death. On one occasion, Aaron tripped over a rock in the garden, and to Deanna it meant that she was to use that particular rock to kill him. When he was playing and throwing rocks at his father and brothers in the yard, she interpreted this as sign of the order in which the boys were to be killed.

Deanna had received many of these strange messages throughout the weeks prior to the month of May. Each time she resisted, the worse the deaths would be for her children. With the increasing pressure of the messages to kill her children, Deanna began preparing. She had remembered the message about the rocks in the garden and decided that this would be the method she would use. She had found the large rock that Aaron had tripped on in the garden and she secretly hid it in his room.

On the evening of May 9, 2003, Deanna went to bed as usual not knowing when God would call on her again. She woke during the night and claimed that she just had a "feeling." In her mind she had received a message stating that "now is the time." Knowing that she had hidden the chosen rock in Aaron's room, she went there first. Aaron, just fourteen-months-old, was lying in his bed sleeping. She picked him up and laid him on the floor. Deanna lifted the rock and hit him with a single blow directly on the head. Aaron began to scream and cry. This immediately woke her husband Keith who was sleeping in the other room. He came running and asked her what was wrong. Deanna assured him that everything was fine and that he should go back to bed, as she pretended to be changing Aaron's diaper. The boy was badly injured, but he was still breathing. She proceeded to place a pillow over his face as he gasped for air. Deanna quietly told God that He would have to finish the job himself. She left him lying on the floor struggling to survive.

Next, Deanna went to retrieve her other two sons. She grabbed Luke first and took him outside to the garden. The only article of clothing that he was wearing was the underwear he went to bed in. She pushed him to the ground and began hitting him repeatedly in the head with a large ten-pound rock that eventually smashed his skull. She pulled him into the darkness of the yard by his feet, hoping that his older brother Joshua would not see him. She placed the same large rock directly on top of his small body.

Finally, she grabbed the oldest of her children, Joshua, who was eight. He struggled and fought his mother with all of his strength. Deanna finally got him to the ground, took another large rock similar to the one she used to kill Luke, and began hitting him in the head. She eventually crushed his skull until he was lifeless. She dragged him into the darkness and placed him next to his brother in the garden.

Immediately afterwards, Deanna called 911. All she said was, "I killed my boys." The police arrived and saw her standing in the garden, blood soaked and completely still. She told them what happened and where she had left Joshua and Luke. Both boys were already deceased and had very serious head injuries. They found the youngest child, Aaron, still alive on the floor in his room. Deanna's husband awoke to find the scene bewildering. He was horrified as to what had happened. His wife was immediately arrested, and young Aaron was taken to the hospital.

In March of 2004, the murder trial of Deanna Laney began. She was charged with two counts of murder in the deaths of her two sons, Joshua and Luke. She was also charged with a single count of injury to a child, Aaron, who survived the attack.

The prosecution opened with their first witness, the 911 operator that spoke to Deanna the night of the murders. The operator stated that Deanna lacked compassion and was oddly straightforward when she said that she had killed her boys. The prosecution explained to the jury that it was their job to decide if she was insane or if she knew exactly what she was doing when she attacked her three children with the rocks.

With obvious similarities to the Andrea Yates case, Joe Owmby of the Harris County District Attorney's Office was consulted. Andrea Yates was the housewife who drowned her five children in the bathtub in 2001. He recommended that the prosecutors retain Dr. Park Dietz as a witness. Dr. Dietz is a world-renowned forensic psychiatrist and was a witness for the prosecution in the Yates case.

In a fifty-minute taped interview with Dr. Dietz, seven months after the killings, Deanna explained how she and Andrea Yates were the chosen ones to kill their children, and they were to be the chosen witnesses after the end of the world. She told him about the time when Aaron was holding the spear and the frog, and that this was a sign of how she should kill them through means of strangulation or possibly stabbing them. Deanna explained to Dr. Dietz how Aaron had tripped over the rock in the garden, and this was a sign from God as to how she should kill the boys. She said that she did not cry or get upset during the killings and the beating of Aaron, as she was only obeying God's demands.

Along with Dr. Dietz, two other forensic psychiatrists were hired. The defense team countered this by hiring another forensic psychiatrist, Dr. Philip Resnick, who had also testified in the Yates trials.

With the psychiatric experts in place, the evaluations of Deanna Laney began. Dr. Dietz was the first to explain his evaluation of her. He described Deanna as being completely delusional at the time of the murders. In his opinion, she had no idea what was right or wrong and that there was no question she was mentally ill. There was, however, no documented proof of a history of mental illness. There were only self-reported incidences of delusions such as her belief about the cause of Aaron's bowel problems and the hallucination of smelling sulfur, which she associated with the devil. Throughout all of the evaluations by the team of experts, they all came to the same conclusion: Deanna was indeed suffering from mental illness at the time of the murders.

However, the jury of eight men and four women still had to look at the facts. Deanna had strategically placed the rock in Aaron's room to be used later that night. She had to convince her husband that she was simply changing Aaron's diaper when he walked in during the first attack. She led each of the older boys out into the garden, one by one, and thought to hide them in the darkness. Deanna also had the clarity to call 911 and tell the operator that she had killed her boys. After her arrest, she told a jailer that she would most likely need an attorney. These facts, along with the expert opinions, all needed to be considered when deciding her fate.

The jury couldn't help but recognize the similarities between the Deanna Laney and Andrea Yates cases. Deanna had mentioned several times that she was a religious sister to Yates. Both housewives were from Texas and were deeply religious. Each woman felt they had no choice but to kill their children, and the same experts were hired in both trials. Laney and Yates both admitted that they had messages from God and were sometimes plagued by the devil. Both women had the clarity to call 911 and explain that they had killed their children.

On April 3, 2004, a jury came to a conclusion after seven hours of deliberation. Despite all of the evidence that could have indicated that Deanna was sane at the time of the murders, she was acquitted of all charges in the deaths of Joshua and Luke and the brutal attack of Aaron. It was found that she was legally insane and was immediately transferred to Vernon State Hospital, a maximum-security facility where medical evaluations could be performed. These evaluations would determine how long it would be before she was released.

Conclusion

In May of 2004, Deanna's husband Keith filed for divorce. In his divorce petition, he requested sole custody of Aaron, who suffers from severe brain damage caused by the beating in 2003. Keith continued to support his wife after the killings and claimed he still loved her. However, he felt that being separated, the difference in personalities, and the incident that occurred had destroyed any chances of reconciliation.

In 2007, Deanna was transferred from Vernon State Hospital to Kerrville State Hospital in Kerrville, Texas. Coincidentally, this is the same hospital where Andrea Yates resides. Laney had been granted unsupervised time away from the hospital by visiting doctors, but the judge in the case put an immediate stop to it. Her defense team tried to appeal this decision, but the Texas Department of Mental Health and Mental Retardation could not grant these privileges to her, even if accompanied by her family.

In May of 2012, Deanna was released from Kerrville State Hospital. The courts concluded that there was no evidence showing that she would commit these crimes again. Only Deanna and her attorneys know where she is.

For many years, Keith Laney had refused interviews, but after the 2012 release of his former wife, he came forward and began speaking out. For many years he has lived with the question of why the mother of his children would commit such a horrific act. After twenty years of marriage, he is still baffled at what suddenly changed and why this happened. He questions why she was released, not knowing if she will harm herself or others after what she did to the children. In his mind, he believes she should still be confined, as most people are not aware of her location, what she's doing, and keeping no record of it.

In February of 2014, Aaron turned twelve. He suffers from severe permanent brain damage. He is absolutely the joy of Keith's life. Unfortunately, witnessing Aaron's hardships is a constant reminder of what his mother took away from him. He has to have his diapers changed every day and he has braces on his legs. He is unable to feed himself, brush his own teeth, or do any other tasks that an average twelve-year-old boy should be able to do.

Keith believes that he must forgive his former wife for what happened to their children. He says that not forgiving will only create bitterness.

Chapter 8: Susan Smith

Background

Susan Smith was born as Susan Leigh Vaughan in Union, South Carolina, on September 26, 1971. Susan was the only child between Harry and Linda Vaughan. Linda was a stay-at-home mom and homemaker, while Harry was a firefighter who later worked in one of the many local Union textile mills. The town of Union was known for growing tobacco, flax, corn, and wheat, as well as its history of hard-working people.

Susan's parents married very young in 1960; Harry was twenty and Linda just seventeen. Linda was pregnant at the time with a child she had conceived from a previous relationship, a son she named Scotty. Later, Linda and Harry conceived Susan and were also raising Scotty as well as another of Linda's sons who was named Michael.

During Susan's childhood, her household became very dysfunctional. Harry and Linda's marriage had many problems. At times, fighting between them became violent to the point where Harry would threaten to kill Linda and himself. To make matters worse, Harry was an alcoholic, which usually was the root of the arguments.

With the tensions in the Vaughan household, Susan and Scotty became very frightened as children. When Susan was pre-school age, her half-brother Scotty unsuccessfully tried to commit suicide by hanging himself. According to her playmates' parents, Susan became a sad little girl around this time.

Although Susan was very sad and had endured much turmoil in the household, she grew up very close to her father. In 1977, when Susan was just six years old, her parents decided to divorce. The split devastated Harry and he quickly became very depressed and began drinking even more heavily.

Just five weeks after the divorce, Harry committed suicide by shooting himself in the abdomen. He was just thirty-seven years old. The suicide had followed an argument between Linda and Harry in which the police were called.

Susan was left with many voids in her life after the death of her father. To complicate the situation, Linda had already remarried just two weeks after her divorce had been finalized. His name was Beverly (Bev) Russell. He was a committeeman for the state of South Carolina as well as a member of the advisory board for the Christian Coalition. The family soon moved into the exclusive Mount Vernon estates section of Union.

In 1987, shortly before Susan's sixteenth birthday, she was sleeping on the sofa one evening. Bev came and sat down at the other end. Susan crawled over, laid her head in Bev's lap, and began to fall asleep. Bev took Susan's hand and moved it towards his genitals. During the molestation, Susan pretended to be asleep. She later told her mother that she did not object to Bev's actions because she wanted to see how far it would go. It was apparent to everyone that Susan's reaction was very inappropriate.

Susan eventually filed a complaint against Bev with the South Carolina Department of Social Services, as well as the Union County Sherriff's Office. Linda contacted Susan's school counselor for guidance. She and her mother only attended counseling sessions four or five times before discontinuing. Charges were never filed against Bev.

Aside from her dysfunctional home life, Susan was excelling in school. When she reached high school, she became a member of the Beta Club, which is a club that requires students to achieve a "B" grade average or better. In 1989, during her senior year, Susan was named "Friendliest Female" at Union High School.

During Susan's junior and senior years of high school, she began working at the local Winn-Dixie grocery store. Without the other employees knowing, she secretly started dating a married coworker. As a result of the affair, she became pregnant and had an abortion. Susan began to date another coworker while the other relationship still existed. The married coworker found out about the second relationship and soon ended their affair. Susan became very upset and depressed over this and in early 1988, she attempted suicide by overdosing with a combination of Tylenol and aspirin. She was admitted to Spartanburg Regional Hospital, and there it was discovered that this was not Susan's first attempt at ending her life. She had apparently taken a similar combination of drugs in excess at the age of thirteen. After a month of recovery, along with the support of the Winn-Dixie managers, Susan returned to work.

David Smith, also a resident of Union, South Carolina took a job at the same Winn-Dixie store as Susan at the age of 16. He was an average student, yet had a very strong work ethic. David and Susan worked together for quite a while and they began to date in the summer of 1990. David had always viewed their relationship as very casual and not at all serious, but in January of 1991, Susan became pregnant. This time, Susan decided to not have an abortion, so she and David married. The marriage gave her a sense of security and stability.

Susan continued working at the Winn-Dixie store until she went into labor, and on October 10, 1991, Michael Daniel Smith was born. Susan and David both continued working at Winn-Dixie, and this soon became one of the sources of tension in their marriage. Shortly after the couple's one-year anniversary, Susan rekindled an affair with her former coworker. This angered David, and in 1992, they separated. The couple went back and forth trying to mend their relationship while living at each of their parents' houses.

In the winter of 1993, David and Susan decided to live under the same roof again, so they bought a house together. Susan soon became pregnant again, and on August 5, 1993, a second son named Alexander Tyler Smith was born. Within 3 weeks of Alex's birth, the couple again decided to separate. In 1994, they finally decided to divorce.

Susan made the choice to change jobs, as she no longer wanted to work at Winn-Dixie with David. She was hired as a receptionist at a company called Conso in Union. Along with work, she had enrolled in some part-time college courses. Susan's workload along with raising her two children soon became too much for her to handle, and things were about to take a very dark turn in her life.

The Lie

October 25, 1994 was like any other day for Susan. She woke the children, fed them, and drove them to the daycare center. Susan went to work as usual and on her lunch break, she decided to join several coworkers for a meal. One of these coworkers was Tom Finley, a man whom Susan was very romantically fond of. While most of her coworkers engaged in conversation, Susan sat without much to say. Around 1:30, Susan decided to ask her supervisor if she could go home. The supervisor asked her why. Susan said that it was because she was in love with someone that wasn't in love with her, referring to Tom. She was allowed to leave, but instead she sat quietly at her desk.

Shortly after 4:30 that afternoon, Susan arrived at the daycare center to pick up her two sons as she did every weekday. After dropping a coworker off at her home, Susan arrived at her own house about 6:00 p.m.

At around 8:00 the same evening, Susan dressed her boys and placed them in their car seats in the backseat of her car. She was very depressed over Tom's rejection and the fact that he only wanted to be friends.

It was close to 9:00 p.m. when a knock at the door startled Union resident Shirley McCloud who lived just a quarter mile from John D. Long Lake. She turned on the porch light and there stood Susan, sobbing hysterically and screaming that she had been carjacked and her children kidnapped. Shirley's husband Rick told their younger son to go call 911. Shirley asked Susan to come into the house so she could talk to her about what had happened. Once she had her calmed down, Susan began to explain the events that led her there.

Susan described the following to Shirley: *"I was stopped at the red light at Monarch Mills and a black man jumped in and told me to drive. I asked him why is he doing this and he said 'shut up and drive or I'll kill you.'"* Susan went on to tell Shirley the direction that the man drove towards. She explained that the abductor made her stop at the sign right near John D. Long

Lake. Susan said she was asked to get out of the car in the middle of the road, and asked him if she could take the kids. The man said that he did not have time and he would not hurt her kids. She said the abductor made her lie on the ground and he then drove away.

The Union County Sheriff's Department began searching for Susan's car, a small Mazda. Sherriff Howard Wells led the investigation and questioned Susan thoroughly. He took notes of Susan's clothing and her disposition. Her face was red and puffy from crying and she sat fairly still with her hands folded in her lap. A police artist later met with Susan and took her description of the black man that allegedly abducted the children and stole her car.

Sheriff Wells called in Chief Robert Stewart who was the head of SLED, or the South Carolina Law Enforcement Division. As Wells began organizing the search, he instructed SLED to coordinate diving efforts in John D. Long Lake. The divers searched the bottom of the lake but didn't find anything. The SLED helicopter also flew over the Sumter National forest and used heat sensors over the lake.

The news media began to descend on Union, South Carolina in large quantities. Radio stations, newspapers, and television crews began covering the carjacking and abduction. David joined his former wife on the steps of the Union County Sheriff's Department and Susan stated the following: *"To whoever has our boys, we ask that you please don't hurt them and bring them back. We love them very much...I plead to the guy please return our children to us safe and unharmed. Everywhere I look, I see their play toys and pictures. They are both wonderful children. I don't know how else to put it and I can't imagine life without them."* After the statement was made, Susan went back to the Union Sheriff's Department where she was questioned further.

On October 27, 1994, two days after the carjacking, Susan and David submitted polygraph tests given by the FBI. David's polygraph results showed that he knew nothing initially about the carjacking or the disappearance of their sons. Susan's test, however, was inconclusive. When she was asked the question, *"Do you know where your children are?"* her test showed a high level of deception. David was only given one polygraph test, but Susan would be given several more in the days to come.

Throughout Susan's interviews, investigators began to see many inconsistencies. She had told investigators that her son, Michael, had asked her to go to Walmart the evening of the carjacking. She said the children were both fussy, so she and her two sons drove over to Walmart, then proceeded to drive to a local park where they sat in the car until 8:40 p.m. Susan described how she drove back to the Walmart parking lot where the light was better, so she would be able to find the baby bottle that Alex had dropped in the backseat of the car. Employees and witnesses from the Walmart were questioned thoroughly and no one saw Susan or her car there that evening. She had also mentioned that they were thinking of visiting a friend named Mitchell that same evening, but when he was questioned about this later, he said he knew nothing about the potential visit.

Investigators became very suspicious of Susan after the interviews and polygraph tests. They continued to press Susan as to why she was inconsistent with her story about being at Walmart and visiting her friend. At one point during an interview, the investigator asked her why her children were fussy that evening, then asked her directly, *"Is this why you killed your children?"* Susan immediately slammed her fist onto the table, stood up, and told the investigator that she couldn't believe he would ask her such a question.

Another person that thought there were inconsistencies in Susan's story was the police sketch artist, Roy Paschal. He had drawn the sketch of the carjacker according to Susan's description. He believed she was overly specific about some details and too vague about others.

The FBI's Behavioral Sciences Unit was called in for assistance to provide a profile of a homicidal mother. The profile, according to the FBI, fit Susan to a T: a woman that grew up in poverty, was in her twenties, had endured sexual abuse, was suicidal, and had experienced rejection from a male recently. The investigators' suspicions were heightened, but there was no hard evidence…yet.

On November 3, 1995, the ninth day after the alleged carjacking and abduction of their sons Alex and Michael, Susan and David prepared for interviews with three separate news networks. The program *CBS This Morning* asked Susan if she had anything to do with the disappearance of her sons. She explained that she had nothing to do with the disappearance of her children, but whoever did was a sick and emotionally unstable person. Even though she and David were not together as a couple any longer, David said he believed his wife.

Susan and David were scheduled for an interview next with the *Union Daily Times*, a local newspaper, but her mother called and cancelled it claiming the two were exhausted and could not make it. Sheriff Wells had contacted Susan earlier and scheduled another interview, but Susan did not tell David or her mother.

At around 1:40 that afternoon, Susan met Sheriff Wells at a small church located near the Union County Courthouse. It was a small meeting room with two folding chairs that sat face to face. Sheriff Wells and Susan sat towards each other, knee to knee. The Sheriff told Susan he knew that her story of the carjacker was a lie. He said that undercover police were around at the location she specified at the time of the carjacking and no signs of trouble were reported. He also told her that he would be obligated to tell the black community of Union of her accusations that a black man carjacked and abducted the children. Susan looked up at Sheriff Wells and asked if he would pray with her. At the end of the prayer he said, *"Lord, we know that all things will be revealed to us in time."* Then he looked up at Susan and told her that it was time.

Susan lowered her head and repeatedly said that she was so ashamed. She asked if she could have Sheriff Wells' gun so that she could kill herself. He asked her why she would want to do something like that. Susan went on to explain that her children were *"not all right."*

Susan began to tell Sheriff Wells about the night of October 25. She said she was consumed with thoughts of suicide as she drove her Mazda along the highway that night. She had planned on driving the boys to her mother's house, but she felt since she was such a failure, her mother would not help her. She was haunted by the thoughts of her abortion and her failed marriage to David. She felt there was no hope. She described how she initially wanted to end all of their lives by placing the car in neutral and allowing it to roll into John D. Long Lake. She had tried twice by pulling on the parking brake, but the car kept stopping. Finally, she stepped outside of the car and released the parking brake, which sent the car rolling over a boat ramp into the lake.

Nine days after the children and Susan's car went missing, Sheriff Wells organized a team of divers from SLED to again secure and search John D. Long Lake. The divers were told the information disclosed by Susan, and shortly after the dive began, the small overturned Mazda was found in eighteen feet of water. The divers peered into the rolled up windows of the car to see two car seats hanging upside down and a small hand that was pressed against the car window. It took nearly an hour to pull the Mazda out of the lake. The windshield was cracked and the car was covered in mud. The bodies of Alex and Michael were taken to the University of South Carolina Medical Center in Charleston for autopsies.

Conclusion

After Susan's confession, she was immediately arrested and charged with two counts of murder in the deaths of her sons. On Friday, November 4, the autopsies were performed and they indeed concluded that the children were alive when their mother sent the car rolling into John D. Long Lake.

In the days that followed her confession, an uproar began throughout the black community of Union and the surrounding areas due to Susan's false accusations that a black man carjacked her and abducted her sons. A local black Minister told the people to pray for healing, not bitterness. Susan's brother, Scotty, made a formal apology on her behalf to the black community through the media and explained that it was not a racial issue.

Susan was held without bail at the York county jail. She was deemed eligible for the death penalty due to the fact that two people were killed in one act, and that they were both under the age of eleven.

On July 11, 1995, Susan's trial began. She had undergone several psychiatric evaluations prior to the beginning of the trial. To the people of Union, she had developed a dual personality, appearing deceitful to most.

On July 27, 1995, after two hours of deliberation, the jury came to the conclusion that Susan should not receive the death penalty, but instead spend the remainder of her natural life in prison. The judge sentenced her to thirty years to life in prison. She will be eligible for parole in the year 2035. She will then be 53 years old.

David Smith, Susan's former husband and the father of Alex and Michael, has since remarried a woman that he met while working at Winn-Dixie and had two more children. He says he still has good days and bad days, the bad usually being around holidays, birthdays, or anniversaries.

Susan is being held in the South Carolina's Leath Correctional Institution near Greenwood. It is said that a former jail mate of Susan's spoke to the National Enquirer in 2013. She disclosed that Susan had paid her to keep an eye out for guards while she was having sexual encounters in the cafeteria and closets with a girlfriend.

Susan's former husband David says that nothing surprises him with Susan. She will do anything to get attention or recognition. She is sneaky and always very convincing and will do what is needed to be in the spotlight.

Chapter 9. Tonya Thomas

Single Mothers

In almost all religions, the birth of a child is considered to be a sacred thing. Be it Buddhism, Christian, Islam, or any other religion, the birth of a child is considered to be one of the greatest miracles sent to mankind by God. It is considered to be a miracle, a gift, a moment of such gratitude and excitement that it alters the lives of people forever. However, as amazing as childbirth really is, there are a number of responsibilities that man must shoulder after the birth of his child. The child's upbringing, teachings, and care all become a parent's responsibility. And perhaps, that is the reason why the norms of society have divided the system amongst two people: the male and the female. In most societies, the male of the house is usually tasked with generating the financial support that is needed for a family to succeed, while the mother is tasked with taking care of the young child.

However, this is what I would call a 'perfect scenario,' something that very few, very lucky people actually have. There are a number of discrepancies that can rise up along the way, the biggest of which is the fact that most people tend to get separated or divorced after a few years. Divorce rates are rising, not only in the United States, but all around the globe. People are looking for new options, moving away from each other. However, they fail to understand the effect this might have on their children. What goes on in the mind of a young child when he finds out that his father and mother, the two people who he has known throughout his life, are now going to be living separately? It is disastrous, to say the least, but really quite common. You personally may know hundreds of cases in which a woman is raising her children alone or a single dad is working away while still raising his children.

Single mothers, of course, find it more difficult to be able to raise the baby on their own and manage their professional lives as well. This becomes difficult and tiresome with one kid, much less four. However, people find ways to deal with their depression and worries, don't they? We resort to drugs, cigarettes, and alcohol in order to 'ease the pain,' even though we know full well that this is never the solution. Rather than alleviating the pain and difficulty altogether by coming to a logical solution, we are just suspending it for a later time. The worrying part is, we become more and more addicted to these things.

Drugs, cigarettes, and alcohol have all been used as reasons for which a lot of people have been killed. They not only suspend our motor abilities, but they also cause a significant reduction in our ability to think properly. In this haze, a man is capable of doing anything, without really remembering what he did. However, in the case of Tonya Thomas, as you will read next, many believe her acts were premeditated, even though she had been drinking. Is there, perhaps, a way by which man can justify the ungratefulness of rejecting the greatest of gifts given to him? A child is a precious being; it needs to be nurtured, cared for, and loved.

Unfortunately, Tonya Thomas was unable to handle those responsibilities, mainly due to her own hardships. This is the story of a mother who committed the worst crime of all: she disgraced the paradigm of motherhood itself.

The Background

An African American mother of four, Tonya Thomas was married to Joe Johnson. Life was happy back then, but things didn't stay that way for long. Reports and court documents reveal that Joe Johnson was a pretty irate husband, often beating Tonya for petty things. For instance, it was mentioned in one of the reports that the young children watched on as Joe Johnson shouted at his wife for not making dinner at all, and then punched her and kicked her until she hit a wall. After this, the children were removed from the household and taken into custody, only to be returned a month later, despite strong objections from the Department of Children and Families.

Joe Johnson had never been a good husband. Just two years before the fatal shootings, Tonya Thomas had filed a complaint regarding domestic violence against her husband. However, just one hearing later, officials dismissed the complaint. It was evident to everybody who lived around the household that things weren't going very smoothly for the family.

Travis St. Peter, a neighbor who lived right next to Tonya Thomas's house, stated that the family was being known across the neighborhood for being quite disruptive, and the sight of a police vehicle was quite familiar at their household. Obviously, this also had an impact upon the children, who became known as 'hoodlums' in the neighborhood, and were seen lighting firecrackers and scaring away the dogs.

The history of the family is filled with reports of domestic violence. Tonya and Joe had four kids: Joel was twelve years old, Jazlin was thirteen, Jaxs was fifteen and the eldest, Pebbles was seventeen years old. Back in April 2012, Jaxs had thrown a bicycle out of a window in the house and had also shouted threatening words to his own mother. The very next day, as Tonya went to wake up Jaxs for school, it is stated in reports that he punched her repeatedly and kicked her as well, prompting her to push him back until a scuffle started.

The neighbors called the police after yells and shouting coming from the house. This is just one of many incidents that happened in the Thomas household.

According to the reports later filed in court by the Department of Children and Families, Tonya was not mentally or verbally abusive towards her children, and the children had also stated that they felt quite safe within their household. The investigators took statements from the neighbors that led them to believe that the children had "bonded well with their parents," and the whole case was signed off on May 13, 2012.

Leading up to the weeks before the fatal event took place, it is unclear as to the amount of contact that the rest of the family had with the man of the house, Joe Johnson. For several months, he had not been living with the family, and according to a report by an investigator on the case, it was apparent that Thomas did not have a relationship with a partner who was supportive of her children and nurturing towards them. This was written in documents just one month before the fatal shootings. There were numerous phone listings for Joe Johnson, which were dialed by an AP reporter on the fateful day, but all of these were either incorrect numbers or were disconnected.

Ultimately, Tonya Thomas was handling immense financial pressures, as well as the pressures of raising her children all on her own. Few could have imagined that she would resort to such drastic measures.

The Murders

The way Tonya Thomas killed her own children is perhaps the most chilling part of the story of all. The murders took place at 4:30 a.m. in the town of Port St. John in Florida. Reports have revealed that at around 3:00 a.m., Tonya sent a message to a coworker that read, "tell my mom what happened, I want to be cremated with my children." This text message is important as it shows that the whole incident was preplanned and she did not kill her four children out of a drunken frenzy.

The whole scenario of the crime is very strange. At 4:30 a.m., the neighbors began hearing gunshots emanating from the Thomas household. A couple of minutes later, two of the children arrived at the doorstep of the neighbors. One of the boys, believed to be Joel, was covered in blood and told his neighbors that his mother had shot them, and they were seeking refuge. Pebbles, the oldest child, was seen walking back towards the household. Then, Tonya stepped out of the house and called the children back inside.

In a report filed by a Brevard County Sheriff Department's spokesperson, witnesses reported Tonya seemed quite calm when she called her children back inside. It is stated that the neighbors called out to the children, telling them not to go into the household, but this report is distorted. As an FBI call later revealed, one of the neighbors is clearly heard yelling, "Get back, you're not getting in our house!"

The police were called to the scene immediately when the kids were seen going back in, and a perimeter was set up around the house. As soon as the police arrived, they heard gunshots within the household. Therefore, rather than penetrating from the front, the SWAT team decided to go in from the back. Pebbles was seen lying in the yard, severely injured from her wounds. She was proclaimed dead soon after by EMTs as she was shifted to the ambulance.

As soon as the SWAT team entered the household, they saw four other bodies, three of which were of the children, and one was that of Tonya Thomas, who had shot herself. Reports later revealed that a total of nineteen shots that had been fired, eighteen of which were directed at the children. Tonya Thomas used a Taurus .38 caliber revolver in order to shoot and kill her four children and herself. One of the children was shot a total of seven times, while the youngest of the children was shot five times at point blank range from a distance of less than two feet away. Two of the children received bullets straight to their chests.

Perhaps the strangest part about the case is the ages of the children. Most of the cases of filicide that we read about occur when a child is at a young age, before the child can really understand what is happening until it is too late. However, the eldest daughter in the household was seventeen years old, which means that she was perfectly capable of sensing the danger. Reports from the neighbors even stated that Tonya was seen outside the household with a gun in her hand, and yet the children walked back inside, which means that they had been accustomed to such acts of domestic violence.

Joe Johnson was later informed of the deaths of his estranged wife and four children, as he had not been living in Brevard County for several months. The murders caused a major psychological impact upon the community of Port St. John, Florida. Three of the children had attended the Space Coast Junior/ Senior High School, and it is believed that Jaxs was a very active kid, loved football and hanging around with his friends. The deaths devastated the entire town.

Since Tonya had killed herself as well, there were barely any investigations and no hearings took place. The case was closed soon after the killings and the children were laid to rest in the local cemetery. Contrary to what Tonya had demanded to her friend in the text message, the children were laid to rest in the Lagrange cemetery. The service was held at the Temple Baptist Church, and lasted around two hours. In the service, people recalled the stories of the children when they had first moved into the neighborhood and first joined the school.

It is a sad ending, to say the least, of what could have been a very different tale for the children, as well as their mother. Jaxs Johnson had loved basketball and Pebbles was a very outgoing cheerleader and loved to hang around with her friends. Despite the violent nature of the children, they were actually fun to hang around with, as stated by the numerous neighbors who attended the service. Unfortunately, things weren't meant to be. The family's Pastor later stated that this was "God's will."

Autopsy reports that were carried out by Dr. Sajid Qaiser revealed that the alcohol content found in Tonya's blood was more than two times higher than the nationally allowed limit, which prompted the investigators to state that the heinous act was perhaps the result of a drunken frenzy. However, as mentioned earlier, a coworker later told a local newspaper that she had sent him a text message regarding her plan.

Analysts later stated that the killings were regarded as "altruistic" by Tonya Thomas, where she began to think that death was perhaps in the best interests of the children. Most would regard it as a horrible crime, but in the mind of Tonya Thomas, she thought that she was doing the children and herself a favor. The story of Tonya Thomas does show a lot of things about the poor standards of society. Each year, between 250 to 300 children are murdered by their own parents for a multitude of different reasons. We can point fingers in numerous directions: poor gun control, lack of help, lack of control and whatnot, but the fact remains that four beautiful young children lost their lives at the hands of the woman who gave birth to them.

Chapter 10: Diane Downs

Background

Diane Elizabeth Downs was born in Phoenix, Arizona on August 7, 1955. Her parents' names were Willadene and Wes Frederickson. Her childhood was pretty standard: she went to school, had tea parties, and made girlfriends. Nothing really seemed out of place. However, she would later claim that her father had molested her when she was a child. Diane studied at the Moon Valley High School and graduated from there soon after. It was there that she met her partner, who became her husband in the near future, Steve Downs. Once high school was over, Diane opted for college at the Pacific Coast Baptist Bible College, which is situated in Orange, California.

Diane studied there for a year until

she got expelled. One day, she was called into her principal's office where she was given an expulsion letter stating that on the grounds of promiscuity, the college had no other option but to expel her. After this, she went back to live with her parents at their home in Phoenix, Arizona. It wasn't long before she hitched up with Steve Downs, and the couple finally married on November 13, 1973. Together, they had three children, Christie Ann (born in 1974), Cheryl Lynne (born in 1976), and Stephen Daniel (born in 1979, and affectionately known as Danny). A year after Danny's birth, Diane and Steve were divorced, after a seven-year marriage.

During the time of her marriage, Diane had gained employment with the United States Postal Service, and was assigned to the mail routes that lay in the city of Cottage Grove, Oregon. Even though it wasn't very obvious to a third party, her friends, family, and neighbors knew that Diane was struggling to raise the children. The neighbors would later tell the police that Diane always prioritized other things before her children. She was also very cruel to her youngest daughter, Cheryl. This news came to light later on, when it was learned that Cheryl had once told a neighbor of her grandparents that she had become very scared of her mother, who was constantly oppressing her and the other children. It was evident that Diane Downs was an unfit parent, but the kids were young at that time, and likely didn't have anyone else to turn to.

The Murders

Nobody really knows why Diane Downs acted the way she did on May 19, 1983, or why she chose to shoot her children. It was a warm, quiet night in Springfield, Oregon when the incident occurred. Even though the night staff at the Mckenzie Willamette Hospital was not expecting any major patients to arrive, they were always prepared. Past experience had taught them that unexpected emergencies could arise at virtually any point in time.

However, nobody could really have anticipated what actually happened that night at approximately 10:48 p.m. There were no warnings, no information on the news, nothing on the radio. It was a silent night until the screeches of car tires filled the air and a red colored late model Nissan with Arizona plates came to a halt right outside the Emergency Room. Dr. John Mackay was the physician in charge, while the two nurses, Shelby Day and Rose Martin, had already gotten off their seats to look out at the person who was shouting outside.

In the driveway stood a blonde woman, somewhere in her twenties, and she kept shouting that somebody had shot her children. Suddenly the whole hospital was up in a ruckus. Professionals from the intensive care rushed out to see what had happened, and a call was made to the police. As soon as Dr. John Mackay saw the children with gunshot wounds, he shouted out to his ER team, explaining the nature of the wounds. Two of the children were still breathing, albeit with much difficulty. The third was lying slumped over on the front seat and there was nothing that the doctors could do to revive her; it was beyond their control. Soon after they wheeled her in, the young child was pronounced dead.

It wasn't until later that the medical team learned the names of the children: Stephen 'Danny' Downs (three years old), Christie Downs (eight years old), and Cheryl Ann Downs (seven years old). The team wasn't concerned with names however. It was the nature of the emergency that mattered. In this quiet, peaceful town, somebody had just tried to murder three beautiful, small children, and they had succeeded with one. The two living children, Christie and Danny, were struggling for their lives. Cheryl had already been pronounced dead. The doctors performed tracheotomies and they were connected to machines that pumped air to their lungs. Despite the severity of their wounds and the nature of their injuries, the two children remained alive.

Soon after police arrived on the scene, Diane's story began to unravel. The entire car and all three children were spattered with blood, but there was no blood on Diane. When the children were brought to the hospital, Danny was suffering from paralysis, Christie had a disabling stroke, and Cheryl Lynn was already dead. Diane Downs herself had been shot in the left arm. What really ticked the police off was the fact that she was a right-handed person, and they immediately suspected that she had shot herself to make the story look more believable.

When they sat her down for questioning, Downs explained she had been traveling through a rural road that ran beside Springfield, Oregon when a "bushy haired stranger" had stopped her. She said that the man shot her and her three children. The investigators who were accustomed to dealing with victims who were suffering from severe trauma after such a horrific incident were immediately suspicious of Diane's story. She wasn't acting like a trauma victim. She wasn't agitated, she wasn't scared, and unlike so many others who had suffered the loss of a child, she wasn't breaking down frequently. After such a traumatic event in a person's life, victims usually take years to recover and a lot of therapy. Instead, Diane remained calm – a bit too calm.

The investigators continued to closely watch Diane Downs, and their suspicions were increased even further when, for the first time after the incident, Diane went to visit Christie Ann, her eldest daughter. What they saw was something very shocking. After suffering from her stroke, Christie was unable to speak, but the expression in her eyes was not one of love, relaxation, or relief. Instead, her eyes became full of obvious fear as her mother approached her, and her heart rate took a massive jump. This was a clear sign for the investigators that Diane had played a role in the shootings of the three children. Yet, they were unable to prove it just yet.

Soon after, investigators also learned that upon arrival at the hospital, Diane had placed a call to a man named Robert Knickerbocker. As information was revealed, it was found that Robert was already a married man, and had studied with Diane during her time in Arizona. It was purported that the two were having an affair. The forensic evidence that later came to light did not correspond with the story laid out by Diane either. The police found no blood on the driver's side of the car, nor any residue of gunpowder on the interior panel of the driver's side or the driver's door. Knickerbocker later came to testify that Diane had been stalking him for quite a while, and that she did not have any qualms about killing his wife, as long as it meant that she was going to have Knickerbocker to herself the whole time. He also stated that he had felt "mentally relaxed" after Downs had departed Oregon, and it allowed him to resolve problems with his own wife. Even though Diane did not explicitly reveal to the police that she owned a .22 caliber handgun, both Steve Downs and Robert Knickerbocker testified that she did, indeed, have a .22 caliber handgun with her.

It was later found that the handgun was bought when she was in Arizona. The investigators were however, unable to recover the original weapon itself, though they did manage to find shell casings at her house. These casings had marks of extractors from the same gun that had been used to shoot the children. The final nail in the coffin was the fact that according to the witnesses, Diane drove the car at a very slow pace towards the hospital, with an estimated speed of around five to seven miles per hour. These statements went directly against Diane's claims to the police that she had sped to the hospital as fast as she could after the shootings. Once this evidence came to light, police filed charges against and arrested Diane Elizabeth Downs on February 28, 1984, nine months after the shootings. She was charged with first-degree murder as well as two counts each of attempted murder and criminal assault.

The evidence had already begun to pile up against Diane long before the trials even began. For instance, she claimed that the killer had waved her down on a lonely road, and thinking that he needed help, she had stopped the car. However, if the killer had wanted the car, would he not have shot the driver – in this case, Diane – first? Since she was the only adult in the car, the killer's main obstacle would be to get her out of the way, not the three children that were huddled in the car. There was really no motive for a "bushy haired stranger" to shoot three young children that posed no threat to him.

One of the biggest obstacles was the fact that Christie Ann had suffered a stroke and was having difficulty speaking. In fact, doctors had advised her not to try to speak at all. The left side of her brain, which controls speech, had been injured. In addition, her left arm had been permanently disabled. Even though Danny had survived the ordeal, doctors said that it was likely he would never be able to walk again.

During the trial, prosecutors stated that Diane had decided to kill the children so she could spend her time with Knickerbocker in complete peace. They were able to recover documents and letters of her correspondences with Knickerbocker, and in one of these letters, he had stated that he did not like children. The last letter from him said that she must not call him back or write him anymore.

In a miraculous turn of events, Christie was able to overcome her injuries and finally started speaking again. During the trial, the nine-year-old was brought to the witness stand, and it was there that she revealed how their own mother had shot the children.

She described the whole event, starting with the family driving from a fast food restaurant along a deserted road, where Diane had parked the car at the side of the road and then got out. She then took out her handgun and shot all three of the children. Christie said that even though she was in immense pain, she saw her mother put the handgun to her left arm and fire a shot as well.

Diane Elizabeth Downs was found guilty on all charges on June 17, 1984 and was given a sentence of life in prison, along with fifty additional years. Psychiatrists who analyzed Downs' condition stated that her personality was very antisocial, and she portrayed narcissistic and histrionic traits as well. While delivering the verdict to the accused, the judge made it evidently clear that he did not want Diane Downs to ever be freed.

One of the prosecutors of the case, Fred Hugi, decided to adopt the two surviving children and they went to live with him and his wife in 1984. Before she had been arrested and tried, Downs was pregnant with a fourth child, to whom she gave birth to just a month after her trial had concluded. She named the girl Amy, but just ten days before she received her final sentence, the State of Oregon seized the baby. Soon after, Amy was adopted by a loving family and renamed Rebecca Babcock, with her nickname becoming Becky.

Drama transpired later on as well, as Downs managed to escape from the Oregon Women's Correctional Center of the

Oregon Department of Corrections on July 11, 1987. Just ten days later, she was arrested in Salem, Oregon. For escaping, an additional five years was added to her sentence. Her sentence allows her to get a parole hearing after having served a total of twenty-five years. Since she is considered to be a dangerous offender, she would be eligible for parole consideration every two years after that first hearing.

In her first parole hearing in December of 2008, Diane proclaimed her innocence by telling her story again. Since she was unable to admit guilt and because her story had now become muddled with different variations of the bushy haired stranger, corrupt law enforcement officials, and strangers wearing ski masks, she was denied parole. She was also denied parole at her next hearing on December 10, 2010. A new law passed recently, which now requires ten years to pass between parole hearings, which means that her next hearing will be held in December of 2020. By that time, Diane Downs will be sixty-five years old, having served virtually her entire life behind prison bars for her heinous crimes.

Epilogue

It is said that the love of a mother for her children is the purest form of love, one of the most natural, purest feelings that exist on this planet. Even though she carries the child for nine months, constantly suffering through severe pain, her love doesn't deter even the slightest. Then, when the child is in his early stages, she feeds him from her breast, cares for him, provides for him, and does everything in her power to make life as comfortable as possible for the little child. She spends her nights devoid of sleep, making sure that the child is properly tucked in and comfortable. If he wakes during the night, she is there to cater to his every need and make sure that the child remains as comfortable as can be.

She cares for the child when he is most vulnerable, protecting him and guiding him away from harm. She does whatever she can to make sure that the child grows up to be an independent, successful being. That is one of the primary reasons why society has granted mothers the highest of positions. In virtually every religion, the sanctity of a mother is highlighted above all others. She is given a much higher status than fathers, and it is natural for a child to call for his mother when he is in pain. It seems as if we were engineered to instinctively call out to our mothers whenever we are in pain or need help.

The question then arises, could this holy figure go against what has been associated with her throughout eternity? Could a mother turn on her child, neglect him and not worry about him? The answer, evidently, is yes. Mothers who become embroiled in drug battles often leave their children to the mercy of this world, not caring about their needs and wants. Then, there are those who leave their children in foster care homes, not caring for a second about the child himself. There are those as well who abort their child, before even giving birth. You will argue that such women do not deserve to be called mothers, and that they should never have been allowed to have a baby. You will say that becoming a mother is a great honor that a woman must fulfill to the best of her capabilities, and if she wants to shun this title, then she is not a good person at all.

Leaving children at foster care homes, deciding to have an abortion, or neglecting the child are some of the things that we have begun to understand over the years. Yes, this happens. We read about it, we watch it on the news, we feel pity, and then we move on. The continuous occurrences of such events have trained our minds to filter out the emotions. Yet, it still hurts when you read about it. The question then begs an answer, what should happen to a mother who decides to kill her own child? What level of punishment should be inflicted on such a person?

RJ Parker

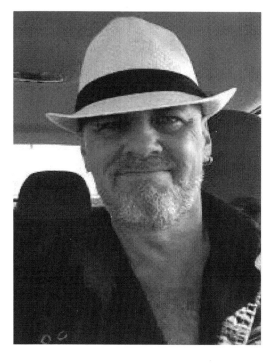

RJ Parker, P.Mgr., CIM, is an award-winning, bestselling true crime author and serial killer expert most well known for his books: *TOP CASES of The FBI*, *Serial Killer Case Files,* and *Cold Blooded Killers*.

Published in 2014 by RJ Parker:

★ Beyond Sticks and Stones: Bullying and Bullycide (March 14)

★ Parents Who Killed Their Children (April 30)

★ Serial Killers Abridged (May 31)

★ Missing Wives, Missing Lives by JJ Slate (June)

★ Social Media Monsters (Internet Killers) (August)

★ Serial Killers True Crime Anthology 2015, Volume 2 (December)

A wide selection of books by Bernard Lee DeLeo is also published by RJ Parker Publishing including: *The John Harding Hard Case* series (4 books), *Rick Cantelli, P.I.* series (2 books), and several action singles as well as YA/Paranormal collections including the *DEMON* trilogy.

RJ was born and raised in Newfoundland and now resides in Ontario and Newfoundland, Canada. Parker started writing after becoming disabled with Anklyosing Spondylitis. He spent twenty-five years in various facets of Government and has two professional designations.

To date, RJ has donated over 1,900 autographed books to allied troops serving overseas and to our wounded warriors recovering in Naval and Army hospitals all over the world. He also donates a percentage of royalties to Victims of Violent Crimes.

If you are a police officer, firefighter, paramedic or serve in the military, active or retired, RJ gives his eBooks freely in appreciation for your service. Please email him.

CONTACT INFORMATION

Facebook:
http://www.facebook.com/AuthorRJParker
Email: AuthorRJParker@gmail.com
Email: Agent@RJParkerPublishing.com
Blog: www.RJParker.net
Website: www.RJParkerPublishing.com
Twitter: @AuthorRJParker

Made in the USA
Middletown, DE
06 May 2018